VISION PATHOLOGY
IN EDUCATION

VISION PATHOLOGY IN EDUCATION

By

EDITH COHOE KIRK, Ed.D.

Adjunct Professor
College of Education
Wayne State University

Illustrated by

JUSTUS W. COHOE

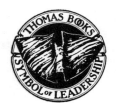

CHARLES C THOMAS • PUBLISHER
Springfield • Illinois • U.S.A.

Published and Distributed Throughout the World by
CHARLES C THOMAS • PUBLISHER
Bannerstone House
301-327 East Lawrence Avenue, Springfield, Illinois, U.S.A.

© *1981 by* CHARLES C THOMAS • PUBLISHER

ISBN 0-398-04505-6
ISBN 0-398-04505-4 (pbk.)

Library of Congress Catalog Card Number: 81-4942

*With THOMAS BOOKS careful attention is given to all details of
manufacturing and design. It is the Publisher's desire to present books that are
satisfactory as to their physical qualities and artistic possibilities and
appropriate for their particular use. THOMAS BOOKS will be true to those
laws of quality that assure a good name and good will.*

Library of Congress Cataloging in Publication Data

Kirk, Edith Cohoe.
    Vision pathology in education.

    Bibliography: p.
    Includes index.
    1. Vision disorders in children. 2. Visually
handicapped children — Education. I. Title.
[DNLM: 1. Ophthalmology — Education. 2. Vision
disorders. WW 18 K59v]
RE48.2.C5K58   618.92′0977′002437   81-4942
ISBN 0-398-04505-6   AACR2
ISBN 0-398-04505-4 (pbk.)

Printed in the United States of America
C-1

FOREWORD

TEACHERS AND OTHERS have been plagued for years with the lack of an adequate textbook which discusses, with a minimum of technical terms, eye physiology and pathology and the relationship of these to education of children. This type of course has been a requirement in curriculums for teachers of visually handicapped children for many years. Textbooks have been general ophthalmology texts or simple adaptations of parts of these books. These have contained substantially more technical information than needed by teachers or, in the case of adaptations, the material is incomplete. One of the most serious shortcomings of these textbooks was lack of explanatory illustrations and educational relevancy. The book *Vision Pathology in Education* substantially remedies these deficiencies.

The question addressed in this book by Professor Edith Kirk is: What should teachers and others who are not physicians know about vision pathologies as these affect education of children? Dr. Kirk draws on her extensive background in the biological sciences as well as her experience in the education of visually impaired children in developing the content of this book.

Readers will especially note the numerous excellent diagrams which make the eye and its pathologies more comprehensible. Laboratory work for students on the dissection of a beef eye, discussion of optics and interpretation of eye reports and educational procedures make this book eminently useful as a basis for learning about eye pathology in the education of children.

KENNETH A. HANNINEN
Teacher Education Division
College of Education
Wayne State University
October, 1980

PREFACE

Vision Pathology in Education is a guide for those who work with children and young persons who have eye defects or diseases severe enough to require special assistance. The book will be particularly helpful for (1) college instructors and (2) special teachers.

College instructors are responsible for providing information on eye pathology to their students, the future teachers of visually impaired children. It is desirable for the instructor to have college courses in anatomy and physiology. Such a background is almost basic to the proper interpretation of material such as this. However, experience in using this book in a college course has demonstrated that if the instructor follows *Vision Pathology* carefully, he or she will have a foundation that is adequate. When used in a college course, the book should be supplemented with models, charts, slides, specimens, ophthalmology books, and professional journals. In addition, Wayne State University has always provided the funds for an ophthalmologist to present a lecture on the latest developments in the field.

It is not necessary to follow the order of this book. However, Chapters 1, 2, and 3 should be covered first so that the reader may have an understanding of the Pathology in Chapters 4, 5, and 6 as well as the Refractive Errors in Chapter 7 and Strabismus in Chapter 8. The instructor may wish to include some pathology as soon as the anatomy and physiology of certain organs are understood. For example, after discussion of the eyelids, ptosis and blepharitis from Chapter 4 may be considered; after an explanation of the lens, cataract and dislocation of the lens from Chapter 6 may be discussed. The instructor may prefer to go directly from Chapter 3 to Chapter 7, Optics and Refraction, and then to Chapter 8, Strabismus. These latter two chapters require considerable explanation.

Chapters 9, 10, and 11 include nontechnical material which

students need in order to apply the principles from the previous chapters in their classroom techniques. Chapter 9, Causes of Visual Impairment in the Schools and Interpreting Eye Examination Reports, lets the prospective teacher know what eye conditions to expect in his or her program, and how to interpret the data in eye examination reports. Chapter 10, Vision Screening During School and Preschool Years, explains the importance of early detection and correction of eye problems, an aid in the prevention of blindness. Chapter 11, Educational Procedures for the Partially Seeing, considers only low visioned children, many of whom are legally blind. This chapter should be helpful for any teacher who has a partially seeing child in the classroom.

The special teacher will use *Vision Pathology* to understand eye problems and their effect on the child. The educational implications mentioned in the book will give the teacher suggestions about how to help the child who has a certain eye condition. The teacher will want to supplement these suggestions by observing the child as he uses his eyes in a variety of learning situations.

As the child progresses in school, the special teacher should give him information about his eye condition so that he continually makes the best use of the vision available to him. This information is necessary as the special teacher guides the child toward his fullest educational potential.

EDITH COHOE KIRK

ACKNOWLEDGMENTS

THE AUTHOR expresses appreciation and gratitude to a number of persons. Dr. Horace L. Weston critically read the entire manuscript and edited the medical material. His many years as an ophthalmologist, his teaching experience at the College of Medicine, Wayne State University, and his work at the School Vision Clinic, uniquely qualify him for such assistance. Justus W. Cohoe, the author's brother, made the line drawings for the publication.

Kenneth J. Mehr, Assistant Chief, Vision Section of the Michigan Department of Public Health, added his expertise to Chapter 10, School and Preschool Vision Testing. Rebecca E. Johnson, a recent student in the Wayne State University course, "Pathology of the Organs of Vision," and now a Braille teacher, read the chapters in order to offer a teacher's viewpoint. Patricia A. Eastland, an outstanding primary teacher in Detroit, critically reviewed Chapter 11, Educational Procedures for the Partially Seeing, to be certain it contained information that the average teacher could understand and use when children and young persons with low vision are in the classroom.

Shirley M. Gustafson, Supervisor of the Program for the Visually Impaired, Detroit Public Schools, furnished statistical material and professional advice. Others assisted substantially in composing this book:

Elma C. Ambrose	Greta A. Leach
John B. Ambrose	Helen M. Maier
Helen N. Blades	Eunice K. Orton
Robert E. Crawford	Edmund Radke
Ann Marie Gangola	Wilma I. Seelye

CONTENTS

xi

VISION PATHOLOGY IN EDUCATION

Chapter 1

ANATOMY AND PHYSIOLOGY

THIS CHAPTER considers the structures and functions of the eye, the orbit, and the accessory organs.

RELATION OF THE BRAIN AND CRANIAL NERVES TO THE ACT OF SEEING

The eye itself is a receptor organ. The act of seeing and interpretation is in the brain at the occipital lobes.

The eyes focus light rays on the retinae; here the rays are converted into nerve impulses. The impulses are carried by the optic nerves and visual pathways to the occipital lobe at the posterior extremity of the brain. At the occipital lobe, the impulses produce the sensation of sight (Figure 1).

Cranial nerves also play a vital part in the act of seeing. Twelve pairs emerge from the under surface of the brain. They are classified as motor (govern muscular movement), sensory (control sensation), and mixed nerves. The nerves are named according to the order in which they arise from the brain and also by names which describe their nature and function.

The following cranial nerves are concerned with vision:

II.	Optic	Sensory	Nerve of the sense of sight
III.	Oculomotor	Motor	
IV.	Trochlear	Motor	Activate muscles of the eye and eyelid
VI.	Abducens	Motor	
V.	Trigeminal	Mixed	Intimately associated with ocular function
VII.	Facial	Mixed	

Thus, half of the cranial nerves are involved with vision. When injury or disease or prenatal conditions affect any of these nerves, trouble with our visual apparatus occurs. The trouble may vary from incoordination to blindness, from trivial to serious disturbances.

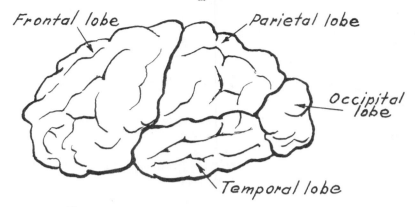

Figure 1. Left side of brain showing occipital lobe.

THE ORBITS AND ACCESSORY ORGANS OF THE EYES

Bony orbits serve as a protection for the eyes. In addition, accessory organs are necessary for both the protection and functioning of the eyes. These are the eyebrow, the eyelids and eyelashes, the conjunctiva, Tenon's capsule, the lacrimal apparatus, and the extraocular muscles.

The Orbits

The orbits are two cavities in the skull situated at the upper and anterior part of the face (Figure 2). They surround the eyes except in the front. Each orbit is shaped like a funnel. The large end of the orbit, directed outward and forward, forms a strong, bony edge which protects the eyeball. The small end is directed backward and inward. It is pierced by a large opening, the optic foramen, through which the optic nerve and ophthalmic artery pass. Other orbital openings permit the passage of additional blood vessels and nerves.

Seven bones assist in the formation of each orbit, but three of these bones are medial and assist in the formation of both orbits. Thus, eleven bones form the two orbits. The bones, which are joined together along suture lines, are covered by a thin tissue called the periosteum.

The eyeball occupies only about one-fifth of the space within each orbit. The contents of the orbit include the eyeball and

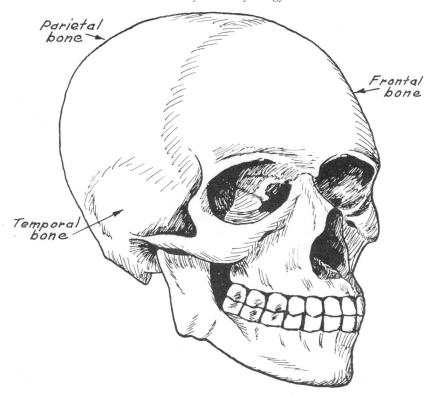

Figure 2. Front view of skull showing orbits.

optic nerve, the ocular muscles, the lacrimal gland, blood vessels, and nerves. Fat fills the spaces between the various structures. Fat and muscle account for the bulk of the other four-fifths of the space within each orbit.

The Accessory Organs

THE EYEBROW. The eyebrow is a thickened ridge of skin that is covered with short hairs and located on the upper border of the orbit. Two main muscles move the eyebrow: the frontal muscle of the forehead raises the brow and the orbicularis muscle of the eyelid lowers it. Thus, the eyebrow controls to a limited extent the amount of light entering the eye. Also, the brow affords some protection against blows directed to the eye.

THE EYELIDS AND EYELASHES. The eyelids are movable folds of tissues which serve to protect the eyes. Each eyelid has four basic layers: skin, muscle, tarsal plate or tarsus, and conjunctiva. The skin of the lids is the thinnest in the body and is freely moveable. The skin continues over the lid margin to fuse with the conjunctiva.

Within the muscle layer the orbicularis muscle encircles the lid opening. The orbicularis muscle closes the lids; in addition, this muscle enables us to squint and blink.

The lids have an almost instantaneous reflex action that causes a blink as a most efficient protective mechanism" (Andrews, 1969, p. 7).

The levator muscle originates at the apex of the orbit and inserts into the tarsal plate of the upper lid (Figure 5). The levator supports and elevates the upper lid.

The tarsal plates or tarsi are thin, elongated plates of dense fibrous tissue which give form and firmness to the part of the lid next to its opening. There are two tarsal plates, one in each upper and one in each lower eyelid. That in the upper is larger than in the lower.

Meibomian glands are long sebaceous glands that are arranged in vertical columns forming yellowish streaks on the inside of the lids (Figure 3). There are about twenty-five on the upper lid and fewer on the lower. They are embedded within the tarsal plates and open on the lid margins. Vaughan and Asbury (1977) state that the meibomian glands produce a sebaceous secretion which forms an oily layer on the tear film. This helps to prevent the rapid evaporation of the tear film.

Eyelashes or cilia are found along the margins of the eyelids. They usually are arranged in two rows curving outward from the surface of the lid. The cilia are provided with sebaceous glands, known as the glands of Zeis. In addition, there are modified sweat glands, the glands of Moll.

The palpebral fissure is the elliptical space which separates the lids when the eye is open. The temporal angle of this space is known as the external canthus and the nasal angle as the internal canthus. The caruncle, a small, reddish elevation of modified skin, is just within the internal canthus. The caruncle helps to

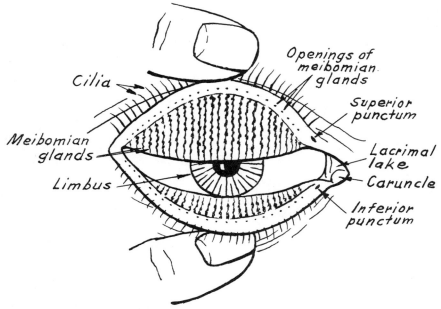

Figure 3. Inverted eyelids showing meibomian glands.

form the lacrimal lake where the tears collect before they are excreted.

The eyelids have a rich blood supply. Scheie and Albert (1969) state that when the lids are injured, this rich blood supply causes them to bleed profusely, but it also facilitates healing and aids in preventing infection.

> The lids protect the eyes from external injury, foreign bodies, undue exposure and excessive light. They serve to distribute the tears and the secretions from the various glands, thus lubricating the eyeball, keeping the surface of the cornea moist and transparent and washing away any dust which may have found its way into the eye (Allen, 1963, p. 33).

THE CONJUNCTIVA. The conjunctiva is a thin, transparent mucous membrane that is divided into two portions: the palpebral and the bulbar. The palpebral conjunctiva lines the eyelids and is firmly attached to the underlying tissue. It is well supplied with blood vessels. The bulbar conjunctiva covers the anterior part of the eyeball except for the cornea. This portion is loosely attached to the sclera except at the limbus where it merges with the epithelium. The loose attachment allows the eye to move freely. Kestenbaum (1963) states that the blood vessels of the bulbar conjunctiva normally do not reach the limbus. Only in pathologic conditions will the conjunctival vessels reach the limbus and invade the cornea.

Mucous secretion from the glands in the conjunctiva furnishes lubrication which allows the lids to move freely over the eyeball.

TENON'S CAPSULE. Tenon's capsule or fascia bulbi is a connective tissue covering of the eyeball. It extends from its fusion with the conjunctiva about 3 mm. behind the limbus, to the posterior pole of the eye where it blends with the sheath of the optic nerve. The sheaths of the extraocular muscles also blend with Tenon's capsule.

Tenon's capsule isolates the eyeball, so as to allow free movement. In wide movements of the eyeball, both the globe and Tenon's capsule move together as a whole upon the surrounding fat in the orbit.

THE LACRIMAL APPARATUS. The lacrimal apparatus has two parts, secretory and excretory. The secretory portion consists of the lacrimal gland. The excretory portion collects the tears and conducts them into the nasal cavity (Figure 4).

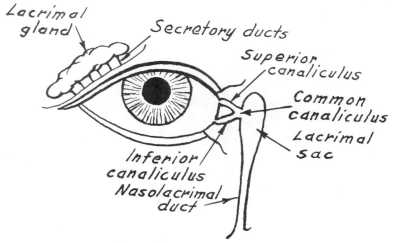

Figure 4. Lacrimal apparatus.

The lacrimal gland is divided into two parts. The larger part, the size of a small almond, lies in a depression in the upper and outer part of the bony orbit. A smaller palpebral portion is contained in the base of the upper eyelid. Tears are constantly being formed in small amounts. Tiny ducts from both portions of the gland pass downward and empty tears over the cornea and conjunctiva. The tears next reach the lacrimal lake near the inner canthus.

The excretory portion of the lacrimal apparatus consists of the puncta, the canaliculi, the lacrimal sac, and the nasolacrimal duct. The puncta are two minute openings, one on the upper lid, the other on the lower (Figure 3). They are on moundlike elevations on the lid margins about 6 mm. from the inner canthus. The puncta siphon tears from the lacrimal lake into the canaliculi. The canaliculi, superior and inferior, are about 1 mm. in diameter and 8 mm. long; they join to form a common canaliculus just before opening into the lacrimal sac. The lacrimal sac is the dilated part of the lacrimal excretory system. The nasolacrimal duct, a downward continuation of the lacrimal sac, opens into the nasal cavity.

> The tears pass into the puncta by capillary attraction. The combined forces of the capillary attraction in the canaliculi, gravity, and the pumping action of the orbicularis oculi muscle on the lacrimal sac tend to continue the flow of tears down the lacrimal duct into the nose and nasopharynx (Vaughan and Asbury, 1977, p. 50).

Vaughan and Asbury (1977, p. 53) give the composition and function of tears. The tears are a mixture of secretions from the lacrimal glands, the goblet cells in the mucous membrane, and the meibomian glands. The tear fluid forms a thin layer that covers the corneal and conjunctival epithelium. The functions of the tear layer are (1) to wet the surface of the corneal and conjunctival epithelium; (2) to make the cornea a smooth optical surface by eradicating minute surface irregularities of its epithelium; and (3) to impede the growth of microorganisms on the conjunctiva and cornea by the mechanical flushing and the antibacterial action of tears. Lysozyme, an enzyme present in tears, can destroy certain bacteria.

Periodic resurfacing of the tear film is important to prevent dry spots and is accomplished by blinking. In the normal eye, blinking maintains a continuous tear film over the ocular surface (Vaughan and Asbury, 1977, p. 54).

The quantity of tears is increased when the eyes are irritated by such factors as wind or smoke, or when the emotions cause us to have tears of joy or sorrow. At such times the drainage function of the lacrimal apparatus is overburdened and the tears spill onto the cheeks.

THE EXTRAOCULAR MUSCLES. The extraocular or extrinsic muscles control the movement of each eye. These consist of four rectus or straight muscles and two oblique. All arise from the wall of the orbit and are inserted into the sclera of the eyeball (Figures 5 and 6).

The four rectus muscles are named according to their approximate positions of placement on the eyeball: superior, inferior, medial, and lateral. All originate at a ring tendon, the annulus of Zinn, at the apex of the orbit. They course forward

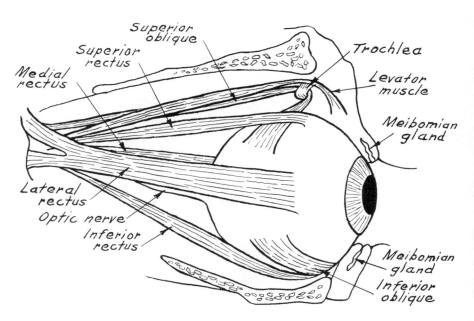

Figure 5. Extraocular muscles and levator muscle, lateral view.

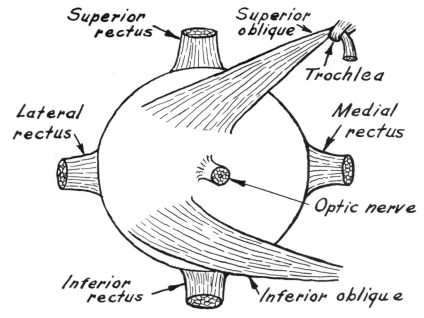

Figure 6. Extraocular muscles, posterior view.

surrounding the optic nerve and diverge as they reach the globe. Each is approximately 40 mm. in length and somewhat ribbonlike. The muscles become tendinous just before their insertion into the sclera. All are inserted in the anterior part of the globe, the distance varying from 5 to 8 mm. from the corneal limbus.

The superior oblique muscle, like the rectus muscles, arises from the apex of the orbit and passes along its nasal wall to the trochlea, a cartilaginous ring, just back of the upper inner angle of the orbit. Here the muscle becomes tendinous. The superior oblique tendon passes through the trochlea and angles outward and somewhat backward to pass beneath the superior rectus to attach to the eyeball. The inferior oblique muscle arises from the lower nasal orbital wall several millimeters behind the orbital rim. It passes back and under the inferior rectus and inserts into the sclera below and slightly lateral to the posterior pole. Thus, both oblique muscles insert on the posterior half of the globe.

Kestenbaum (1963) notes that the extraocular eye muscles have special features that separate them from other muscles.

Their fibers are thinner and are not united in bundles that are separated by connective tissue, and they have more nerve fibers than do other muscles.

The extraocular muscles are innervated by branches of the third cranial nerve, the oculomotor, with the exception of the lateral rectus and superior oblique. The lateral rectus is supplied by the sixth nerve, the abducens, and the superior oblique by the fourth nerve, the trochlear.

The four rectus muscles acting singly turn the corneal surface upward, downward, inward, or outward as their names suggest. The action of the two oblique muscles is complicated, but their general tendency is to roll the eyeball on its axis.

The extraocular muscles are able to move the eyeball about 45 degrees in any direction except down, where the movement increases to 60 degrees. This is helpful because most of our work is done in a downward gaze (Andrews, 1969).

> If it is remembered that under-action of any one of the twelve muscles involved in all ocular movements may produce diplopia, it must be admitted that the perfect functioning of these muscles represents a degree of precision which the most exacting engineer will admire (Martin-Doyle, 1951, p. 171).

THE COATS OR TUNICS OF THE EYEBALL

The eyeball is spherical in shape except in the front, and is about one inch in diameter (Figure 7). It consists of three coats; from the outside inward, these are:

> The fibrous coat: cornea and sclera
> The uveal tract (vascular coat): iris, ciliary, body, and choroid
> The neural coat: retina.

The Fibrous Coat

THE CORNEA. The cornea is the anterior, transparent portion of the fibrous coat, covering one-sixth of the eyeball. The cornea is continuous with the sclera which overlaps it, as a watch crystal is overlapped by the case into which it is fitted. The junction where the cornea and sclera meet is known as the limbus (Figures 3 and 9).

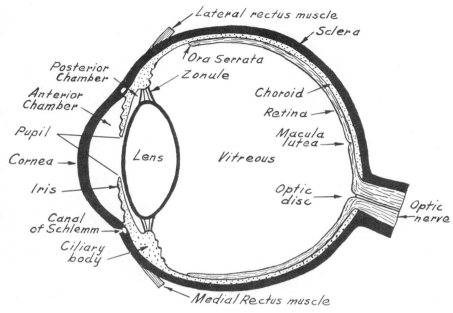

Figure 7. Horizontal section of right eyeball from above.

The cornea is about 1 mm. thick and has five layers (Figure 8). From anterior to posterior, these are: (1) epithelium, (2) Bowman's membrane, (3) stroma, (4) Descemet's membrane, and (5) endothelium.

The epithelium covers the front of the eye and is five or six cell layers thick. Bowman's membrane is a clear, acellular layer that supports the epithelium and acts as a barrier to protect the underlying stroma. Bowman's membrane is a modified layer of the stroma to which it is firmly adherent. If destroyed, Bowman's membrane does not regenerate; instead, corneal epithelium fills the defect.

The stroma, the thickest layer of the cornea, is formed of connective tissue. Descemet's membrane is a thin, firm layer which consists of many fibers. It is developed from the endothelial cells and can regenerate from them. Descemet's membrane is elastic and is more resistant than the remainder of the cornea to trauma and disease. The endothelium consists of a single layer of cells.

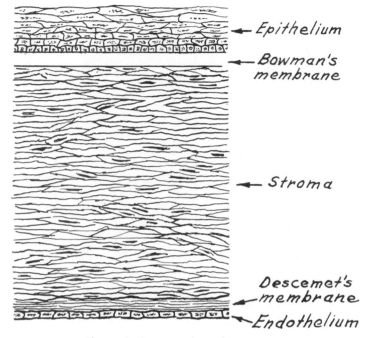

Figure 8. Cross-section of cornea.

Chemical or physical damage to the endothelium of the cornea is far more serious than epithelial damage. Destruction of the endothelial cells may cause marked swelling of the cornea and result in loss of its transparency. On the other hand, damage to the epithelium causes slight and transient localized swelling of the corneal stroma which clears following rapid regeneration of the epithelial cells (Vaughan and Asbury, 1977, p. 86).

The cornea is clear and avascular with a tear layer covering its surface. Its nutrients are supplied by blood vessels of the limbus, by aqueous fluid inside the eye and by oxygen from the air. The cornea has many nerve fibers which come from the fifth cranial nerve, the trigeminal. Thus, severe pain results from seemingly minor irritations.

The cornea is not only a protective layer, but also a refractive one. In fact, the chief refraction of light rays occurs at its surface. Vaughan and Asbury (1977) state that the cornea has a refractive power equivalent to a plus 43 diopter lens. Its anterior surface has two-and-one-half times the focusing power of the lens. Any change in the shape or transparency of the cornea interferes with the formation of a clear image.

The tear film which covers the surface of the cornea and moistens the lining of the eyelids, maintains the proper optical qualities of the cornea. A reduced production of tears may result in injury to the cornea and impaired vision.

THE SCLERA. The sclera is the posterior, opaque portion of the fibrous coat, covering five-sixths of the eyeball (Figure 7). It is continuous with the cornea at the limbus anteriorly and with the external fibrous sheath of the optic nerve posteriorly. (The part of the sclera through which the nerve passes is known as the lamina cribrosa.) Around the optic nerve the sclera is penetrated by blood vessels and nerves.

The sclera is approximately 1 mm. thick, but varies at different points. It is composed of three layers; from anterior to posterior these are: (1) outer or episclera, (2) sclera proper, and (3) inner lamina fusca. The episclera is a filmy, elastic, and highly vascular connective tissue that separates the sclera proper from Tenon's capsule and the conjunctiva. The sclera proper is white, strong, and inelastic. It is composed of bundles of connective tissue with some elastic fibers. Though traversed by many blood vessels, the sclera itself is relatively avascular; it receives nutrients from the blood vessels of the episclera. The inner lamina fusca is a brown pigment layer that is united by filaments of connective tissue to the choroid.

The sclera maintains the shape of the eyeball. It supports and protects the delicate inner structures of the eye.

The Uveal Tract (Vascular Coat)

The uveal tract lies immediately beneath the sclera and cornea and is protected by them (Figure 7). It runs from the pupillary border to the optic nerve and is composed of three parts: iris, ciliary body, and choroid. These three parts have a close and continuous relationship one with the other; this accounts for the frequency with which pathology involves the whole of the uveal tract. The function of the uveal tract is to nourish the eyeball.

THE IRIS. The iris is a thin, colored membrane circular in form, located just behind the cornea (Figure 7). It has an opening in the center, the pupil, through which light is admitted to the eye chamber. The iris is an anterior extension of the ciliary body and is connected to the sclera and cornea at the limbus. Except for this attachment at the circumference, the iris hangs free in the anterior of the eyeball.

In structure the iris consists of a delicate, spongy connective tissue stroma containing a rich supply of blood vessels, pigmented cells, muscles, and nerves. Scheie and Albert (1969, p. 57) state that normally the anterior surface of the iris has no lining. The posterior surface of the iris contains two layers of pigmented epithelium; this prevents the entrance of light.

There are two sets of muscles in the stroma of the iris, the sphincter and the dilator. The sphincter, which consists of a narrow band of tissue about 1 mm. wide, encircles the pupil. Its function is to constrict the pupil. The dilator muscle runs radially from the circumference of the iris to the pupil. It dilates the pupil.

The function of the iris is to control the amount of light entering the eye and thus assist in obtaining clear images. The regulation is accomplished by the action of the sphincter and dilator muscles. The sphincter muscle contracts, diminishing the size of the pupil when the eye is stimulated by a bright light or is looking at a near object. The dilator muscle contracts, increasing the size of the pupil when the light is dim or when the eye is looking at a distant object. Pupillary size is also influenced by drugs, vascular filling, and psychic factors.

When the iris is cut the elasticity of the blood vessels closes them. Thus, almost no blood escapes except at the base of the iris. A congested iris may bleed. Ordinary incisions or cuts of the iris, except at the base, produce almost no bleeding so no clotting is produced. Clotting is necessary for scar tissue healing. A hole or cut made in the iris will not ordinarily close by scarring as do other wounds. This is a valuable asset in many types of eye operations.

THE CILIARY BODY. The ciliary body is that part of the uveal tract that extends backward from the root of the iris to the anterior margin of the choroid (Figure 7). It forms an asymmet-

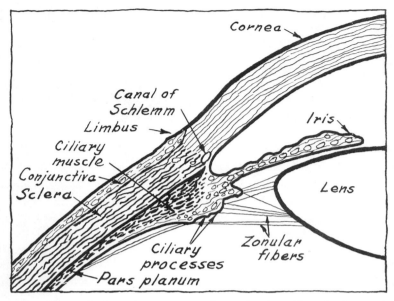

Figure 9. Anterior segment of eye showing ciliary body.

rical band about 6 mm. long and has two main parts, the ciliary processes and the ciliary muscle (Figure 9). In longitudinal section, the ciliary body is triangular in shape with the base facing toward the iris and the apex merging with the choroid. The inner side of the triangle forms the ciliary processes at the anterior portion and the flat part, pars planum, of the ciliary body at the posterior portion. The outer side of the triangle forms the ciliary muscle.

The ciliary body is well supplied with blood vessels and nerves and has at least six layers, including two layers of epithelium, that cover the ciliary body on its inner surface.

The ciliary processes are made up of approximately 70 villus-like processes about 2 mm. long and arranged so as to form a circle behind the iris. They are composed mainly of capillaries and veins. The epithelium of the ciliary processes secretes aqueous, a nutrient fluid, into the interior of the eye. The zonule which holds the lens in place, originates in the valleys between the ciliary processes.

According to the Helmholtz theory of accommodation, contraction of the ciliary muscle relaxes the zonular fibers, releasing the tension on the elastic lens capsule, and allowing the lens to become more spherical. This increases the refractive power of the eye and enables focusing on near objects. Relaxation of the ciliary muscle returns the tension to the zonular fibers and the lens assumes its original shape. (Accommodation will be discussed further when the lens is considered.)

THE CHOROID. The choroid is the posterior portion of the uveal tract extending from the ciliary body to the entrance of the optic nerve (Figure 7). It is firmly attached to the margin of the optic nerve. The choroid varies in thickness from approximately .15 mm. to .22 mm.

The choroid is largely composed of blood vessels united by delicate connective tissue containing pigment cells and nerve fibers. There are three layers of blood vessels in the choroid. These vessels are largest in the external layers and become smaller as they reach the inner layers, eventually forming a fine capillary network, the choriocapillaris. External to the blood vessel layers is the avascular suprachoroid which loosely attaches the choroid to the sclera; internal to the vessel layers is the structureless Bruch's membrane.

The choroid's function is to nourish the outer layers of the retina, the vitreous, and lens. It serves to conduct nerves and blood vessels to the anterior part of the eye. It is thought that the pigment of the choroid absorbs excess light that enters the eye.

> The degree of choroidal pigmentation varies considerably. Negroes, Asiatics, and other heavily pigmented people tend to have deeply pigmented choroids. Lightly pigmented people with blond hair and blue eyes tend to have lightly pigmented choroids (Scheie and Albert, 1969, pp. 61-62).

Summary of the functions of the uveal tract:

> The function of the iris is to control the amount of light which enters the eye. This occurs by reflex constriction of the pupil under the stimulus of light and dilation of the pupil in darkness. The ciliary body forms the root of the iris and serves, through the zonular fibers, to govern the size of the lens in accommodation. Aqueous humor is secreted by the ciliary processes into the posterior chamber. The choroid consists of abundant blood vessels; its function is to nourish the outer portion of the underlying retina (Vaughan and Asbury, 1977, p. 107).

The Neural Coat

The retina, the innermost layer of the eye, is a delicate nerve membrane (Figure 7). It receives the images of external objects. Impressions made by these objects are transferred to the occipital lobe, the center of sight in the brain. All the other structures of the eye exist only to nourish and protect the retina and to focus light rays upon it.

The retina covers two-thirds of the inner surface of the globe. Anteriorly it extends nearly to the ciliary body where it terminates in a jagged margin, the ora serrata. Posteriorly it is continuous with the optic nerve attached to it. The retina is 0.1 mm. thick at the ora serrata and 0.23 mm. at the posterior pole. It is thinnest at the fovea centralis, area of clearest vision.

The retina is firmly attached to a layer of pigment epithelium both at its anterior border and at the optic nerve. Between these two points the retina is in contact, but not firmly attached to the pigment epithelium.

There are nine layers in the retina proper (Figure 10). The layer next to the pigment epithelium contains the light receptor elements, the rods and cones. The inner layers are occupied by conducting elements, bipolar and ganglion cells and supporting elements. The layer next to the internal limiting membrane has only nerve fibers which converge to form the optic nerve.

At the center of the posterior part of the retina, corresponding to the axis of the eye, is the yellow spot, or macula lutea (Figures 7 and 11). In the center of the macula is the fovea centralis. This is the region of most distinct vision and contains only cones. In the fovea the innermost layers (of retina) are thinned to allow less interference with the transmission of light rays.

About 3 mm. to the inner side of the macula is the head of the optic nerve, known as the optic disc. The disc is the only part of the retina from which the power of vision is absent; for this reason it is called the blind spot.

Except at the macula, rods are more numerous than cones (Figure 10). The rods are narrow cylinders which consist of two portions, an outer and inner. The outer segment contains visual purple or rhodopsin which bleaches with light. The inner seg-

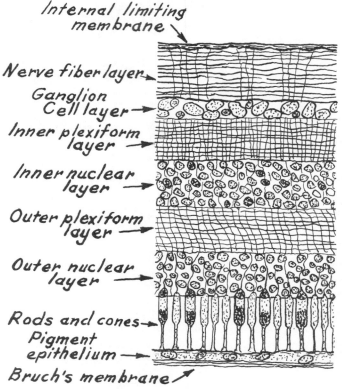

Internal limiting
    membrane

Nerve fiber layer

Ganglion
    Cell layer

Inner plexiform
    layer

Inner nuclear
    layer

Outer plexiform
    layer

Outer nuclear
    layer

Rods and cones

Pigment
    epithelium

Bruch's membrane

Figure 10. Cross-section of retina.

ment is slightly thicker. The cones are conical or flask-shaped, and like the rods, are composed of two portions, an outer and inner. The cones in the macula are long cylinders, appearing much like rods.

Light must traverse most of the retinal layers in order to activate the rods and cones. The light stimulus is absorbed by the pigment epithelium and passes to the rod or cone-cell nucleus, and down the axon to communicate with the dendrite of the bipolar cell in the outer plexiform (network) layer. The bipolar cell then transmits the impulse by means of its axon to the dendrite of the ganglion cell in the inner plexiform layer. The axons of the ganglion cells assemble in the nerve fiber layer and join to form the optic nerve.

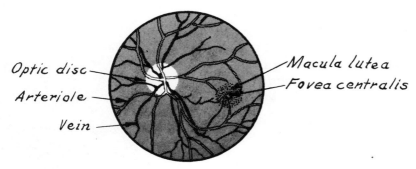

Optic disc
Arteriole
Vein

Macula lutea
Fovea centralis

Figure 11. Fundus showing disc and macula.

Rods function best in dim light; this is known as scotopic vision. The rods give night vision and visual orientation; they also detect movement. Thus the rods make it possible to walk without tripping over objects that are seen as hazards even though they are not clearly seen. A driver's rod vision will first detect a car approaching from a side street.

Cones function best in bright light; this is called photopic vision. The cones give detailed vision, such as for reading or for distinguishing distant objects; they also provide color vision. When the driver's rod vision detects an approaching car, he will turn his eyes so that the foveal cones may discern the details of the vehicle.

The retina does not have pain fibers. Loss of vision, either central or peripheral, is likely to indicate retinal pathology. The retina receives its blood supply from two sources: (1) the central retinal artery, which enters through the optic nerve, supplies the inner two-thirds of the retina; and (2) the choriocapillaris of the choroid, which provides the outer third, including the fovea.

The choriocapillaris is the only blood supply to the fovea. Thus, when the retina is detached, the fovea is liable to irreversible damage.

THE OPTIC NERVE AND OPTIC TRACT

The optic nerve, the second cranial nerve, is the pathway for the sense of sight (Figure 7). It is formed of axons of the ganglion cell layer of the retina. These fibers converge to form the optic disc, the beginning of the optic nerve, an oval area at the posterior part of the eye.

The disc is named from its appearance when the eye specialist uses an ophthalmoscope to examine the interior of a patient's eye, the fundus (Figure 11). The disc serves as the principal landmark during the eye examination, and is the only part of the central nervous system that can be seen.

The optic nerve leaves the eye from the back of the globe through a circular opening in the sclera. Behind the globe the

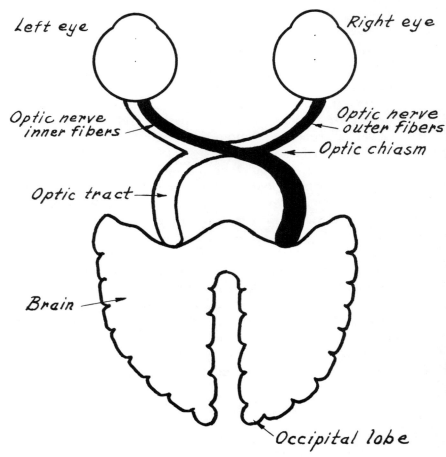

Figure 12. The optic chiasm.

optic nerve is covered by the same three layers that encase the brain. This orbital portion of the nerve which is about 25 mm. long, lies loosely in order to permit free range of movement of the globe. The central retinal artery and vein enter the optic nerve about 10 mm. behind the globe. The presence of these blood vessels in the optic nerve gives an abundant supply of blood to the optic nerve fibers.

The optic nerves from both eyes pass backward through the optic foramina, openings in the skull. Just posterior to the optic foramina, in the brain cavity itself, the two nerves come together, and the fibers from the inner portions cross (Figure 12). This is known as the optic chiasm and is an incomplete crossing of fibers, since the outer fibers do not cross. The crossed fibers join the uncrossed fibers of the opposite side to form the optic tracts. Each tract then goes to the lateral geniculate body, oval prominences on the forebrain, just posterior to the chiasm. Here the fibers connect with a new set of nerve fibers that extend back to the occipital lobe of the brain. Both the visualization of an image and the interpretation of what is seen, occur in the brain itself.

CONTENTS OF THE EYEBALL

Within the eyeball are the aqueous humor, the lens, and the vitreous body (Figure 7). The aqueous is a specific body humor, the lens is an anatomical structure, and the vitreous is a gel-like mass. There are three chambers within the eye: the anterior and posterior aqueous chambers and the vitreous chamber. The iris separates the anterior and posterior chambers. The anterior chamber lies in front of the iris; the posterior chamber is between the iris and the lens. The two chambers communicate through the pupil space of the iris.

Aqueous Humor

Aqueous humor fills the anterior and posterior chambers of the eye (Figure 7). It is a clear, watery fluid which is similar in composition to blood serum, but contains almost no protein. Its function is to nourish the anterior portion of the eyeball, especially the cornea, lens, and part of the vitreous.

Aqueous is secreted by the ciliary body into the posterior

chamber of the eye. It passes slowly through the pupil space into the anterior chamber. The aqueous next passes through the trabecula, a meshwork located at the junction of the iris with the sclerocorneal region. Finally it leaves the eye through the circular canal of Schlemm which lies within the sclera, and the anterior ciliary veins. This constant flow of aqueous into and out of the eye normally maintains intraocular pressure at about 20 mm. of mercury.

> The intraocular pressure is determined by the rate of aqueous production by the ciliary body epithelium and the resistance to outflow of aqueous from the eye (Vaughan and Asbury, 1977, p. 214).
>
> The aqueous humor is constantly being formed, and constantly eliminated from the eye, and the rate of production and absorption are so nicely balanced that under normal conditions the intraocular pressure is kept at a relatively constant level. Anything which upsets this level, such as an increase or decrease in either formation or absorption, will result in a change in intraocular pressure unless both processes undergo an equal and simultaneous change (Adler, 1962, p. 331).

The Lens

The lens is a biconvex, transparent structure about 4 mm. thick and 9 mm. in diameter, lying directly behind the iris (Figures 7 and 9). It is located between the aqueous fluid and vitreous body. The lens is enclosed in an elastic membrane or capsule that is very resistant to chemical influence.

Beneath the anterior lens capsule is a layer of epithelial cells. These cells become elongated until, finally, at the equator proper, they are long and thin. The equatorial cells produce lens fibers throughout the life of the individual. As new cells are formed, they move toward the center of the lens and become more compact. The outer fibers which form the cortex are much softer than the inner fibers, the nucleus. The lens changes shape throughout life due to lens fiber growth and uneven or unbalanced swelling and shrinking in later years.

The zonule, which originates in the ciliary processes, holds the lens in place by means of its delicate but strong fibers (Figures 7 and 9). The fibers insert into the lens capsule close to the equator, and extend around its circumference.

The lens does not have pain fibers, blood vessels, or nerves. It is nourished by the aqueous.

The function of the lens is to focus light rays upon the retina. Accommodation takes place when focusing on a near object, one within 20 feet of the observer: the ciliary muscle contracts, pulling the choroid forward and releasing tension on the zonule. This permits the lens to become more convex, thus increasing its power. When the eye is at rest or focusing on a distant object (20 feet or more away), the ciliary muscle relaxes and the zonular fibers are taut, exerting a pull on the lens that flattens its surface.

> The changes produced in the lens by age are the following:
> In the foetus its form is nearly spherical, its color of a slightly reddish tint, it is not perfectly transparent, and is so soft as to break down readily on the slightest pressure.
> In the adult the posterior surface is more convex than the anterior; it is colorless, transparent, and firm in texture.
> In old age it becomes flattened on both surfaces, slightly opaque, of an amber tint, and increases in density (Pick and Howden, 1977, p. 841).

The Vitreous

The vitreous is a clear, transparent gel-like body that occupies about two-thirds of the interior of the eyeball, lying between the lens and the retina (Figure 7). Like the cavity which it fills, the vitreous is spheroid with a saucer-shaped depression into which the lens fits. The vitreous is quite impervious to cells and debris.

The outer surface of the vitreous has a hyaloid membrane; this is not a true membrane, but a condensation of the gel at its surface. The vitreous has a firm attachment to the pars plana epithelium and the retina immediately behind the ora serrata. In the normal eye the vitreous contains no fixed cells, blood vessels, or nerve fibers. It receives its nourishment from the surrounding tissues: the choroid, ciliary body and retina.

The vitreous maintains the form of the eye, and gives support to the structures within the eye. Since it is quite impervious to cells and debris, the vitreous assists in sustaining the transparency of the eye.

REFERENCES

Adler, Francis H. *Textbook of Ophthalmology.* 7th ed. Philadelphia: W. B. Saunders, 1962.

Allen, James H. *May's Diseases of the Eye.* 23rd ed. Baltimore: Williams and Wilkins, 1963.

Andrews, Edson J. *Synopsis of Ophthalmology*. Tallahassee: Florida State University, 1969.

Kestenbaum, Alfred. *Applied Anatomy of the Eye*. New York: Grune and Stratton, 1963.

Kronfeld, Peter C. *The Human Eye in Anatomical Transparencies*. Rochester: Bausch and Lomb Press, 1943.

Martin-Doyle, J. L. C. *A Synopsis of Ophthalmology*. Bristol, England: John Wright & Sons, 1951.

Pick, T. Pickering and Howden, Robert, (Eds.). *Gray's Anatomy*. 15th ed. New York: Bounty Books, 1977.

Scheie, Harold G. and Albert, Daniel M. *Alder's Textbook of Ophthalmology*. 8th ed. Philadelphia: W. B. Saunders, 1969.

Vaughan, Daniel and Asbury, Taylor. *General Ophthalmology*. 8th ed. Los Altos: Lange Medical Publications, 1977.

Chapter 2

DISSECTION OF A BEEF EYE

IT IS STRONGLY recommended that at the completion of Chapter 1, Anatomy and Physiology, the students examine and dissect a beef eye. Even though charts, models, and various texts have been used, this experience is a high point of the course. Students have a much better understanding and appreciation of the human eye if given the opportunity to dissect a beef eye.

Before the dissection the students should bring the following equipment:

> Scissors, 5-inch with a fine point preferred
> Forceps
> Single-edged razor blades
> Magnifying glass or lens
> Disposable plate or dish at least 6 inches in diameter in which to place the eye
> A small glass or plastic dish for floating the lens and vitreous.

The instructor supplies the beef eyes, water, paper towels, and newsprint. Fresh eyes, one for each student, should be obtained. The eyes may be kept in a freezer until two or three hours before dissection. This will allow time for thawing.

IDENTIFICATION OF OUTSIDE STRUCTURES

The fat and extraocular muscles are cut away from the outside of the eye, leaving the optic nerve. The students will then observe the following:

> The thin, transparent conjunctiva
> The spherical shape of the eyeball
> The cornea fitting onto the sclera as does a crystal on a watch
> The greater curvature of the cornea as compared with that of the sclera

27

The horizontally oval shape of the pupil and its surrounding iris

The fatty, whitish appearance of the optic nerve.

IDENTIFICATION OF INSIDE STRUCTURES

The eyeball is sectioned by inserting the scissor point and cutting around the circumference half-way between the front and back. While this is being done, aqueous from the anterior and posterior chambers will escape.* When the front half of the eyeball is lifted off, the lens and vitreous can be removed intact. The students will notice the following:

The difficulty of cutting through the sclera because of its toughness

The transparency of the cornea

The iris and its attachment at the limbus, but otherwise hanging free

The anterior chamber from which part of the aqueous escaped can be identified by inserting scissors or forceps between the iris and cornea

The ciliary body which extends backward from the iris and surrounded the lens before it was removed

The thinness of the choroid layer because of the absence of blood

The tapetum, the bluish area in the choroid, which some animals have for seeing in the dark

The very thin neural layer of the retina which has become detached except at the optic disc

The optic disc which marks the beginning of the optic nerve inside the eye

The lens, observing how it fits into the saucer-like depression in the vitreous

The clear, gel-like vitreous body held together by an invisible membrane.

---

* "At the equator of the eyeball one is not entering either the anterior or the posterior aqueous chamber, but the trauma of handling and incising will probably have allowed the aqueous to escape into the vitreous chamber" (Weston, 1979, p. 6).

The lens and vitreous may be floated in water. The lens can carefully be pulled free; this is difficult because of the tiny zonular fibers that hold it in place. Comparison can then be made of its anterior and posterior surfaces, noting that the anterior surface is more curved. The lens is placed over newsprint in order to observe its magnifying power. The capsule surrounding the lens can now be removed, leaving a shapeless, jelly-like mass.

REFERENCES

Havener, William H. *Synopsis of Ophthalmology.* 4th ed. St. Louis: C. V. Mosby, 1975.

Schut, A. L. *Anatomy and Physiology of the Human Eye.* Kalamazoo: Western Michigan University, Undated.

Weston, Horace L. Unpublished notes to the author, 10 p., 1979.

Chapter 3

GROWTH OF THE EYE AND DEVELOPMENT OF VISION

A T BIRTH the eye is large and is a functioning sensory organ. Early in life the eye reaches near adult proportions.

The eye is an outgrowth of the forepart of the brain and its growth parallels that of the brain. The greatest amount of growth of the brain and eye takes place during the first year, and continues at a rapid rate until three years of age. Then growth continues at a slower rate until approximately fourteen years of age. Thereafter little growth occurs. The eye has reached its adult size by the time of puberty.

DEVELOPMENT OF THE STRUCTURES OF THE EYE

In general, the structures of the anterior part of the eye grow proportionately much less than do those of the posterior.

> At birth the anterior portion of the eyeball has reached almost its adult size; the posterior portion undergoes most of the postnatal increase in size (Weston, 1979, p. 4).

The Sclera

The sclera of the newborn baby is thin and translucent; the bluish color is caused by the blood vessels in the underlying uvea. As its fibers thicken, the sclera becomes more opaque and the eye assumes a glistening, white appearance.

The Cornea

The cornea is relatively large at birth and reaches adult size at approximately two years of age. As the anterior part of the eye grows, the cornea may be molded into a different shape. During the first four to seven years of life there is a tendency for the vertical meridian to become more curved than the horizontal. This is likely to result in astigmatism.

30

The Iris

At birth there is little or no pigment on the anterior surface of the iris. Most newborn infants have bluish irides caused by the posterior pigment layer showing through the translucent tissues. The color deepens as pigment is formed on the anterior surface during the first few months of life. By six months of age, the physician usually knows whether the eyes will become brown or remain blue.

The pupil is small at birth as a result of the poorly developed dilator muscle of the iris. The dilator muscle does not acquire its adult power until five years of age. The pupil is largest from five years through adolescence.

The Ciliary Body

The infant's ciliary muscle has little ability to accommodate. During the first five years of life many new muscle cells are formed, increasing the range of accommodation. This greater range makes it possible for older children to see in detail an object which is no more than 3 inches from the eyes.

The Lens

At birth the lens is nearly spherical. It grows in size throughout life. The new fibers are added to the periphery; this makes the lens of an older person flat or disc shaped. From birth to puberty the lens mass doubles, but thereafter the growth rate slackens.

The Retina

The macula of the infant does not fully develop until four to six months of age. Ophthalmoscopically the fundus of the infant at 6 months is similar to that of an adult.

GROWTH OF THE ORBIT AND ACCESSORY PARTS OF THE EYE

The Orbit

At birth the orbital opening is almost round with the walls being close to the eyeball. Subsequent growth and development of the skull give the opening a roughly square shape. The eye is then more loosely placed within the orbit. There is a great increase in the orbital volume; it is more than doubled during the first year of life and quadrupled by the sixth year.

Growth of the orbit normally continues until puberty. However, decrease in volume of orbital content, as in childhood enucleation or microphthalmos, does not provide the normal stimulus for full development of the bony orbit.

The Palpebral Fissure

There is an increase in the horizontal dimension of the palpebral fissure, from approximately 18 mm. at birth to 30 mm. at maturity. About half of the growth takes place by four years of age.

The Lacrimal Apparatus

The lacrimal gland is somewhat underdeveloped at birth; it reaches its full growth by three or four years of age. Usually the infant does not have tears during the first few weeks of life. However, there is enough tear production to moisten the mucous membranes and the cornea.

The nasolacrimal duct between the tear sac and the nose usually opens at birth.

CHANGES IN REFRACTION WITH GROWTH

The infant eye is short in axial length and is normally 2 or 3 diopters hyperopic.

> About 80% of children are born hyperopic, 5% myopic, and 15% emmetropic. Hyperopia increases until about 7-8 years of age and then gradually decreases until 19 or 20 years of age. After age 7 or 8, myopia gradually increases until about 25 years. (Hyperopia decreases much less than myopia increases.) (Vaughan and Asbury, 1977, p. 13).

GROWTH OF MONOCULAR VISION

The newborn infant has sufficient eye structure to permit a crude visual reflex. However, the layers which encase the optic nerve and visual pathways are not complete, and the rods and cones are incomplete at birth.

The newborn does not have sharp central vision because the macula is not developed. The paracentral vision probably does function to some extent so the newborn does see what is in front of him, but vaguely.

During the first days or weeks of life, the infant shows erratic, uncoordinated movements of the eyes. Lid movements of the same nature occur. The infant does not have the protective blink reflex in response to a threatening visual stimulus until approximately two months of age.

Evidence of central vision is shown by central fixation and by following the object of regard. There is a weak following movement of the eyes at five or six weeks of age. This is shown when a bright object, such as an examining light, is held close to the eyes and moved slowly. By 3 months of age this reflex is well developed to the right, left, up, and down. However, the infant is not yet able to converge the eyes while following an object which is moving toward them.

> At approximately 4 months, macular fixation begins to be associated with hand movements that grasp for the fixation target. As soon as the grasping maneuver succeeds, the target is brought to the mouth and examined by the lips, tongue and gingiva. Therefore, the 4-month-old infant depends upon vision to detect and localize the target, but really upon the mouth to identify and acquaint himself with it. Two more months will pass before the infant transfers these functions completely to his visual reflex and abandons his mouth for this purpose (Parks, 1966, p. 22).

Steady foveal fixation gives a visual acuity of 20/20 or better to the average child seven years of age or older, providing he has a sharply focused image on the fovea and is attentive.

DEVELOPMENT OF BINOCULAR VISION

The development of binocular vision parallels that of monocular vision. To have fusion, there must be binocular vision. Fusion is present consistently by six months, and is firmly established by twelve months. After the child reaches seven years of age, the fusion reflex is matured and is difficult to alter.

MATURATION OF ACCOMMODATION

At the age of four to six months, the infant is able to accommodate. By this age the foveal reflex has become established, and the ciliary muscle has gained strength.

Convergence of the visual lines and pupillary constriction are usually associated with accommodation although they do not always accompany that function. Each of these phenomena can act independently or in greater or lesser association with the others. They can be demonstrated to be present at six months of age.

REFERENCES

Parks, Marshall M. "Growth and Development of the Eye and the Development of Vision." In Sumner D. Liebman and Sydney S. Gellis (Eds.), *The Pediatrician's Ophthalmology.* St. Louis: C. V. Mosby, 1966, 15-25.

Vaughan, Daniel and Asbury, Taylor. *General Ophthalmology.* 8th ed. Los Altos: Lange Medical Publications, 1977.

Weston, Horace L. Unpublished notes to the author, 10 p., 1979.

Chapter 4

DISEASES AND DEFECTS OF THE EYEBALL, ORBIT, EYELIDS, LACRIMAL APPARATUS, AND CONJUNCTIVA, AND THEIR EDUCATIONAL IMPLICATIONS

THIS CHAPTER and the following two will discuss diseases and defects of the eyeball as a whole, the orbit, and accessory organs; also, the coats of the eye and its contents. Educational implications will be considered.

THE EYEBALL AS A WHOLE

Anophthalmos

Anophthalmos is a congenital condition in which one or both eyeballs are absent or rudimentary. The defect is usually bilateral. The orbits are typically small. Eyelids are usually present, but they are concave and small.

As with most congenital ocular defects, anophthalmos is genetically determined, or it may be caused by interference with the development of the embryo. Scheie and Albert (1969) state that drugs, for example thalidomide, may induce this eye condition. Infants with anophthalmos are likely to have multiple defects of the eyes and body.

Educational Implications

Parents of an infant with anophthalmos should have the services of a teacher-consultant soon after the baby's birth. Since the child will have no vision, not even light perception, he will need much help in acquiring daily living skills.

Microphthalmos

Microphthalmos is a condition in which one or both eyes are smaller than normal. Usually both eyes are involved. Microphthalmos is nearly always genetically determined, but may be caused by a prenatal intrauterine infection, such as rubella.

In microphthalmos the eye appears normal, but is only about two thirds the regular size. The affliction may be associated with other ocular defects, such as high hyperopia, aniridia, and cataracts as well as certain somatic abnormalities, for example, club foot and cleft palate (Vaughan and Asbury, 1977). Because of its small size, the microphthalmic eye has a tendency to glaucoma.

There is no treatment for microphthalmos, but the eyes should be checked frequently for signs of glaucoma.

Educational Implications

In Detroit there are usually some children with microphthalmos in the special classes for the blind. These children and their parents need the services of a preschool teacher-consultant. Their main avenues of learning are their auditory and tactile senses supplemented by vision when possible.

Only rarely does a child with microphthalmos have enough vision to be educated in the program for the partially seeing, using such aids as large type, special lighting, and magnifiers.

Glaucoma

Glaucoma is characterized by an increase in intraocular pressure. The increased pressure causes pathologic changes in the optic disc and defects in the visual field. In the open-angle type which comprises at least 90 percent of the cases, there are no symptoms in the early stages. Open-angle glaucoma is insidious, developing so gradually that unless detected by routine testing, it is likely to become well established before being apparent to the subject. Meanwhile the subject has gradually lost peripheral vision which cannot be restored. However, if treatment is started early enough, the ophthalmologist can usually stop the progress of the condition. Untreated glaucoma results in severe visual loss or blindness.

Glaucoma may start at any age. At the present time about 2 percent of the population over forty years of age has glaucoma (Vaughan and Asbury, 1977). This group is urged to have a medical eye examination, including a test for tension, at least every two years.

Increasing numbers of physicians are using the ophthalmoscope to examine the optic disc* of their patients for changes associated with glaucoma, and the tonometer to determine their intraocular pressure. Questionable patients are then referred to an ophthalmologist for treatment.

Primary glaucoma is unrelated to other ocular diseases. It is divided into open-angle or chronic simple and angle-closure or narrow angle glaucoma. Congenital glaucoma is a primary type. Secondary glaucoma results from other ocular diseases and defects.

OPEN-ANGLE OR CHRONIC SIMPLE GLAUCOMA. This type of glaucoma is bilateral and genetically determined. The cause is an obstruction in the drainage apparatus at the trabeculum, the canal of Schlemm, or the ciliary veins. The degree of obstruction generally is related to the elevation in pressure.

Findings

Weston (1979) gives the following findings. Open-angle glaucoma has no definite early symptom. The intermittent, dull headaches which may be present when the pressure is elevated are not distinguishable from those of eyestrain or many other forms of headache. Unless it is detected by actual measurement of the intraocular pressure (tonometry), the condition is likely to become far advanced before the subject realizes that he has trouble. The early damage is loss of vision in parts of the visual field which are off-center enough that they are not noticed. Field losses are due to destruction of nerve fibers which accompanies the development of cupping of the optic disc. As the disease advances, peripheral vision fades, abnormal blind spots develop just outside the central vision area and, lastly, the central vision is lost.

Treatment

The object of therapy is to assist the outflow of aqueous from the trabeculum and the canal of Schlemm. The treatment is primarily medical. Miotics, medications that constrict the pupil,

---

* "Disc changes are extremely difficult to evaluate because of the diversity of normal variations in disc anatomy" (Weston, 1979, p. 6).

facilitate aqueous outflow. At the present time pilocarpine is the drug commonly used. Epinephrine is another drug used because it decreases aqueous production and also increases the aqueous outflow.

Prognosis

The prognosis of open-angle glaucoma is considered good when the drugs are used as prescribed, and when the glaucoma has not already caused extensive damage.

ANGLE-CLOSURE GLAUCOMA. Angle-closure glaucoma has both chronic and acute forms. The chronic form may or may not have acute episodes and may behave much like open-angle glaucoma (without symptoms) for many years before its probable diagnosis through an acute attack. This discussion will be concerned only with the acute form.

Acute angle-closure glaucoma is likely to occur in eyes with shallow anterior chambers and short axial length. The root of the iris comes in contact with the trabeculum and cuts off the outflow of aqueous. The intraocular pressure then rises causing severe pain and sudden loss of vision.

Findings

The symptoms of acute angle-closure glaucoma are quite different from those of open-angle glaucoma. There is a sudden onset of blurred vision, headache, severe pain in the eye, and halos may be seen around lights. Nausea and vomiting are common. Other findings include markedly increased pressure, swollen cornea, fixed dilated pupil, and decreased visual acuity.

It is thought that a factor precipitating the attack is pupillary dilation which permits the iris root to sag forward and close the angle. Stress and excitement, including emotional upsets, may increase the aqueous flow and thus assist in overburdening the trabeculum.

Treatment

Medical treatment is first used to reduce the pressure. If the pressure does not begin to fall in four to six hours, surgery must be done. Peripheral iridectomy is the procedure commonly used. In this operation a portion of the periphery of the iris is excised. A direct channel is formed through the iris for the aqueous to flow from the posterior to the anterior chamber. The same operation is often performed on the other eye to prevent another acute attack.

Prognosis

Usually peripheral iridectomies result in a cure if permanent anterior adhesions have not formed.

INFANTILE GLAUCOMA OR BUPHTHALMOS. Infantile glaucoma is a disease of the infant or very young child. Typical signs are present at birth or in the first three years. Infantile glaucoma is nearly always bilateral and is more common in boys than girls (Martin-Doyle, 1951). It is inherited through a recessive gene. The disease is caused by a congenital defect in, or a blockage of, the angle where the aqueous leaves the anterior chamber to enter the canal of Schlemm and the venous system. As in other types of glaucoma, the aqueous does not drain normally and there is an increase in intraocular pressure.

Findings

The earliest symptoms are tearing and photophobia. The increased pressure results in glaucomatous cupping, a concave depression of the optic disc. Also, since a child's tissues are less rigid than those of an adult, the pressure stretches the corneal and scleral tissues. The cornea becomes hazy, its epithelium swells, and ruptures appear in Descemet's membrane. The anterior chamber increases in depth. This is associated with the enlargement of the cornea and sclera, and has led to the term "buphthalmos" or ox eye.

Treatment

The usual surgical treatment is goniotomy in which the abnormal tissue blocking the anterior chamber is incised. This procedure controls the intraocular pressure permanently in the majority of uncomplicated eyes. Medical treatment is useful mainly to reduce the tension and clear the cornea so that surgery may be performed with precision. When no treatment is given, the eye keeps stretching and may even rupture. Blindness is the result.

Prognosis

The general opinion among ophthalmologists is that even though the tension can be controlled permanently, the long-term visual results are not good.

> The earlier the disease becomes manifest, the less favorable the prognosis, since the early appearance of symptoms implies a more severe defect of aqueous drainage (Vaughan and Asbury, 1977, p. 223).

Educational Implications

At the present time 6.5 percent of the children in the Detroit program for the blind have infantile or congenital glaucoma. Only occasionally is such a child able to progress in a program for the partially seeing.

The irritability and restlessness which these children may show is undoubtedly caused by the pain and frustration which they have experienced.

SECONDARY GLAUCOMA. Glaucoma that follows as a result of some ocular disease or abnormality is known as secondary glaucoma. The ophthalmologist periodically measures the pressure of (1) those subjects with eye pathologies that are known to produce secondary glaucoma and (2) those on topical steroid therapy. Such steroids may produce secondary glaucoma especially if the subject is known to have glaucoma or a family history of it, or if he is given systemic corticosteroids over a long period of time.

Among the eye pathologies that may produce secondary glaucoma are iridocyclitis, dislocation of the lens, intraocular tumors, and trauma. The elevated pressure normally occurs because of increased resistance to aqueous outflow. The resistance may be brought about by some obstruction such as blood cells or pigment in the trabeculum, injury to the trabeculum, adhesion of the iris to the cornea (anterior synechia) or to the lens (posterior synechia), atrophy of the iris, detachment of the choroid, and a production of too much aqueous.

Treatment consists of drugs to reduce the aqueous secretion.

With higher elevations, osmotic drugs are prescribed to prevent permanent damage to the vision while or until the underlying cause of the glaucoma can be treated.

> The secondary glaucomas occur in conjunction with some recognizable ocular disease which leads to the pressure elevation. The causes of secondary glaucoma are numerous, and many are poorly understood. The relative rarity of some of these conditions makes this study very difficult. As a group, however, they represent some of the most severe and hard-to-manage glaucomas. Experimental production of these conditions in laboratory animals is a major need and should be strongly encouraged (Becker and Kolker, 1967, p. 111).

Educational Implications

Since visually handicapped children frequently have more than one serious eye problem, occasionally some develop secondary glaucoma. Such glaucoma may not appear until the youth is in junior or senior high school. Special teachers should make strenuous efforts to be certain that such young persons have annual eye examinations that include tonometry, and follow-up procedures.

Special teachers report that young persons with secondary glaucoma may tire by afternoon, especially after extensive use of their eyes. Also, severe headaches sometimes precede this type of glaucoma.

Occasionally children with glaucoma require prescribed eye medication instilled during the school day. Usually either the child himself or the school administration assumes this responsibility.

Nystagmus

Nystagmus is defined as involuntary, rhythmically repeated movements of one or both eyes. The movements are most often horizontal and both eyes are generally affected. Nystagmus may usually be described as either jerky or pendular.

In jerky nystagmus, movements in one direction are usually relatively slow followed by rapid return to the original position. This type is usually associated with internal ear, neurological, or drug intoxication problems.

Alcohol intoxication, barbiturates, Dilantin,™ and inflammation of the brain in encephalitis also can lead to central nystagmus. Nystagmus that follows ingestion of toxic amounts of a drug ordinarily relents as the drug is metabolized. Malnutrition complicates the picture in chronic alcoholism, frequently necessitating general supportive measurements including vitamin supplements before the nystagmus relents (Scheie and Albert, 1969, p. 326).

When nystagmus commences in adult life, the subject may experience dizziness and annoyance from the apparent movement of objects.

In pendular, often called ocular, nystagmus the movements are of equal speed, size, and duration in each direction. Its most common causes are congenital impairment of vision in the eye or optic nerve, or defective vision in the first years of life. Such defective vision may result from corneal opacity, high astigmatism, aniridia, congenital cataract, bilateral macular lesions, albinism, coloboma of the optic disc, or optic atrophy.

In each condition an incomplete or defective set of visual impulses is transmitted to the brain, preventing the development of the normal fixation reflexes, and pendular nystagmus of ocular derivation occurs. If vision is lost after the second year of life, ocular nystagmus develops in a partial or abortive form. If vision is lost in adulthood, the eyes often are stable (Scheie and Albert, 1969, p. 326).

Congenital nystagmus is hereditary, but many cases are sporadic. The subject may adopt a tilted head position in order to obtain the clearest vision; also, he may show head nodding. The usual infantile cases of nystagmus cannot be treated, though the condition sometimes decreases with advancing years.

Educational Implications

Children or young persons with nystagmus as their primary eye defect comprise 14.6 percent of the enrollment in the program for partially seeing and 13.0 percent in the program for the blind. Many partially seeing children adjust to nystagmus and do much better than expected from their visual acuity tests and eye reports.

If vision can be improved appreciably or eyestrain reduced by eyeglasses, they should be worn. Any assistance, however slight, should be used to ease reading and writing. Also, the child should be allowed to adopt head turning since this is the result of experiencing least disability at that attitude. Any attempt to correct head turning must certainly increase nervous tension.

Children with nystagmus need relief from having to do close eye work for long periods of time. Writing at the chalkboard instead of at their desks provides a pleasant change. Listening to tapes and records and typing from dictation give relief, while increasing the amount of material the children can assimilate.

Young children with nystagmus often show more head movement than others. They may have trouble in keeping the place in the book. Bookmarks used above the line are helpful. The use of the bookmark should be discontinued if (or when) the child no longer needs it. These children fatigue quickly and usually read efficiently for only a short period.

The act of reading, writing, and other near point activities are laborious for children and young persons with nystagmus. Thus, they may need to remain in the special education program longer than do certain other visually impaired students.

Occasionally a young partially seeing child with a progressive eye disease, such as retinitis pigmentosa, also has nystagmus that is accompanied by head nodding. The energy that he uses in reading and writing is tremendous and certainly causes tension and frustration. The school system should consider transferring such a child to a program for the blind where his eyes are no longer the main avenue of learning.

Blind children with nystagmus usually have other severe eye pathology and thus, if they have a small amount of vision, are not expected to be dependent upon it for school progress.

THE ORBIT

Exophthalmos

Exophthalmos is the abnormal protrusion of the eyeball. It may be unilateral or bilateral. Since the orbit is an enclosed, bony space, except at the anterior opening, any increase in the quantity of contents can only push the eye forward. Among the causes of exophthalmos are tumors, systemic disorders, inflammations, fractures or hemorrhages, and congenital orbital anomalies.

Thyroid disease may cause exophthalmos that is either uni-lateral or bilateral. Benign tumors most frequently cause ex-ophthalmos in children. Congenitally shallow orbits and mal-development of the cranial and facial bones may result in protrusion of the eyeball.

If the eyeball is pushed forward rapidly, ocular movements may be disturbed and double vision results. In addition, if the eyelids can no longer protect the cornea adequately, there may be pain from exposure followed by injury to the cornea.

The treatment of exophthalmos must be directed against the cause.

Enophthalmos

Enophthalmos is a backward displacement of the eyeball into its bony socket. Its most common cause is injuries which involve fractures of the wall or floor of the orbit. However, the condition may be present at birth. When congenital, enophthalmos is likely to be bilateral and associated with other congenital defects, such as microphthalmos and ptosis.

Educational Implications

Enophthalmos in association with microphthalmos is likely to result in very low vision. Teacher-consultant service should be given the parents. When such a child enters school, he is likely to need to be educated as a blind child using Braille reading and writing materials. Orientation and mobility training will enable him to know more about his environment and how to move about in it.

Orbital Cellulitis

Orbital infections are seldom primary; instead, they come from the bloodstream infection of adjacent structures, or pene-trating (orbital) injuries. The source of the infection may have only a minor effect on the subject while the orbital inflammation results in severe symptoms (Scheie and Albert, 1969, p. 202).

Orbital cellulitis occurs mostly in young children and fre-quently causes exophthalmos. The onset is often sudden. Other findings are ocular pain, swelling and redness of the lid, swelling of the conjunctiva, and a reduction in ocular movement. The subject is very ill and has a fever.

Treatment is by antibiotics; usually large doses are required. This is necessary in order to prevent such complications as corneal ulcer, optic nerve atrophy, and a posterior extension of the infection.

The visual prognosis is considered to be excellent unless there are complications.

THE EYELIDS

Ptosis

Ptosis is a drooping or prolapse of the upper lid. It is one of the common anomalies of the lid, and may be either inherited as a dominant trait or acquired.

Hereditary ptosis is usually congenital, but may not have its onset until later.

In most instances it is bilateral. Congenital ptosis usually results from a developmental failure of the levator muscle, alone or in association with a weakness of the superior rectus muscle, and occasionally with anomalies of other extraocular muscles.

Acquired ptosis may be caused by a lesion in the pathway at any part of the third cranial nerve, the oculomotor, that innervates the levator muscle. Ptosis may result from an eyelid that is too heavy (because of a swelling or tumor, for example) for a normal levator muscle to lift. In addition, ptosis appears as an early symptom in myasthenia gravis and as a later one in muscular dystrophy.

Findings

The drooping lid of congenital ptosis is quickly noticed. The affected lid is smooth and flat and does not show the normal tarsal fold. If the lid partly covers the pupil, the child is likely to tilt his head and lift his brow in an attempt to see; this causes the forehead to wrinkle. When the lid completely covers one pupil, amblyopia from disuse may develop.

Treatment

The doctor must first find the direct cause: a specific disorder of the muscle(s) or nerve(s), a tumor, or a general disease.

Surgery is the usual treatment for congenital ptosis and is generally done when the child is three or four years old. However, if the ptosis causes obstruction of vision, surgery may be necessary earlier. Surgery consists of shortening the levator muscle when it is not completely paralyzed. Otherwise, an attachment must be made between the frontalis muscle of the forehead and the tarsus of the eyelid, thereby raising the lid as the brow is raised.

When ptosis is caused by a tumor or a general disease, treatment must be concerned with the cause.

Prognosis

Surgery for treating congenital ptosis is quite successful, although occasionally it is necessary to do more than one operation to achieve equal openings for the eyes (Scholz, 1960, p. 75).

Educational Implications

Most children with corrected ptosis do not need to enter special education but can make normal progress in the regular school program. However, occasionally there is a child in the Detroit classes for the partially seeing who has ptosis as his primary eye difficulty.

As these children do their school work, they should be permitted to assume a head position that is comfortable and enables them to have maximum vision.

The special teacher should be alert for children in the school population who have ptosis but have not yet been referred to an ophthalmologist. Referral and follow-up are necessary for cosmetic reasons and for attaining the best possible vision for the child.

Blepharitis

Blepharitis, an inflammation of the lid margins, frequently occurs in children. The condition is usually bilateral and chronic. There are two main types of blepharitis. Seborrheic, the more common, is caused by a functional disturbance of the sebaceous glands which results in an increased discharge; this is likely to be associated with seborrhea of the scalp, brows, and ears. The staphylococcal type is caused by the staphylococcus bacteria and is usually ulcerative. Often both types are present at the same time (Vaughan and Asbury, 1977, p. 46).

The following factors are thought to contribute to blepharitis: general debility, malnutrition, lack of sleep, and uncorrected refractive errors, especially hyperopia.

Findings

The lid margins have a red appearance and are irritated and itching. Scales cling to the base of the lashes in both the upper and lower lids. In the seborrheic type the scales are greasy and the lid margins less red. In the staphylococcal type, the scales are dry and ulcerated areas appear along the lid margins, causing patchy loss of lashes. Conjunctivitis, mild keratitis, and chronic meibomianitis are present.

Treatment

Scales must be removed from the lid margins daily and the scalp, eyebrows, and lid margins kept clean with soap and water in the seborrheic type of blepharitis. Antibiotics or sulfonamide eye ointment is used in the staphylococcal type. Contributing factors such as nutrition, sleep, and correction of refractive errors are part of the treatment. When the two types of blepharitis are mixed, they may run a chronic course for months or even years if not treated adequately.

Educational Implications

The special education teacher, when called upon or as needed, should work with the parents of a child with blepharitis to be certain that contributing factors are being checked: evaluation of the general health, optimum nutrition, correction of refractive errors, and referral for further ophthalmological care.

Hordeolum

Hordeolum is a staphylococcal infection of glands in the eyelid; it may be external or internal. External hordeolum, or sty, is an infection of the lid glands of Zeiss or Moll. The sty is localized and points to the skin side of the lid margin. Sties are more common in children and young adults than in the general population. Persons with refractive errors or blepharitis are more susceptible to sties than are other people. Recurrence is common.

Internal hordeolum is an infection of a meibomian gland. This type is more painful than the sty because of the pressure buildup within the fibrous tissue. Internal hordeola usually point to the conjunctival portion of the lid but may point to the skin side.

Findings

The first symptom may be photophobia, lacrimation, and a foreign body sensation. The area affected becomes red, swollen, and very tender. Vaughan and Asbury (1977, p. 45) state that the primary symptom is pain and its intensity is in direct proportion to the amount of lid swelling. Internal hordeolum affects a larger area and is usually more severe.

Treatment

Treatment of both types of hordeola consists of warm compresses and local antibiotics. (These antibiotics serve only to suppress spread of infection to the conjunctiva and adjacent meibomian glands.) In addition, subjects should be checked for refractive errors and associated blepharitis. All of these measures will decrease the tendency for hordeola to recur.

Educational Implications

Since hordeola are linked with a lowered state of health, the special teacher may need to assist the parents to follow through on the correction of refractive errors and in the treatment of blepharitis, if present.

The special teacher should try to prevent a child with a sty from touching or rubbing his eyes. Cleanliness is important. When a child has an eye infection that the teacher suspects may be spread to others, this information should be reported to the school principal or administrative personnel.

LACRIMAL APPARATUS

Defects of the lacrimal gland and drainage system, especially congenital ones, are relatively rare. Only the most common one, dacryocystitis, will be considered here.

Dacryocystitis

Dacryocystitis is an inflammation of the lacrimal or tear sac. It is almost always associated with an obstruction of the nasolacrimal duct and is generally unilateral. This disease commonly occurs in infants and in persons over forty years of age (Vaughan and Asbury, 1977, p. 50). Only the infant form will be discussed here.

In infants the cause of dacryocystitis is the failure of one of the nasolacrimal ducts to open before birth or during the first few weeks of life. The condition is usually chronic and tearing is the chief symptom.

Treatment consists of massaging the nose region above the tear sac and instilling antibiotic or sulfonamide drops. If this does not stop the tearing after a few weeks, probing the nasolacrimal duct is the procedure used by the ophthalmologist.

One probing is effective in the great majority of subjects. Occasionally repeated probings are necessary to bring about a cure.

THE CONJUNCTIVA

Conjunctivitis

Conjunctivitis is an inflammation of the conjunctiva. Chalkey (1974) considers conjunctivitis the most universal of all eye diseases, while Vaughan and Asbury (1977) state that it is the most common one in the Western Hemisphere.

Some forms of conjunctivitis are very mild causing only redness of the eye and tearing, while other forms may cause great destruction unless treated promptly. Occasionally the source of conjunctivitis is within the body, but usually it is from outside. Because of its exposed position, the conjunctiva is subject to many airborne agents: bacteria, viruses, dust, pollen, fungi, parasites, allergies and chemical irritations. However, the conjunctiva is quite resistant to the effects of all of these.

Many factors tend to make most conjunctivitis a self-limiting disease.

> —tears, abundant lymphoid elements, constant epithelial exfoliation, a cool conjunctival sac due to tear evaporation, the pumping action of the tear drainage system (unimpeded when the lids are open), and the fact that bacteria are caught in the conjunctival mucus and then excreted (Vaughan and Asbury, 1977, p. 60).

There are many symptoms and signs of conjunctivitis. These may include a feeling that something is in the eye, a burning sensation, itching, redness of the eye, tearing, exudation, drooping of the upper lid, and even the formation of a membrane.

BACTERIAL CONJUNCTIVITIS. Bacterial conjunctivitis is the most common form. Staphylococcus, Streptococcus, Pneumococcus and Haemophillus are some of the bacteria causing this disease. This type of conjunctivitis can be either acute or chronic, and the acute types may become chronic.

Findings

Bacterial conjunctivitis makes the eyes red, congested, and irritated. There is a purulent exudate which causes the lashes to be stuck together on waking. Infections by different kinds of bacteria vary in intensity.

Acute catarrhal conjunctivitis or "pink eye" causes the eye to become exceedingly inflamed and produce a moderate discharge.

Treatment

The specific treatment of bacterial conjunctivitis depends on the particular agent responsible. While waiting for the results of laboratory tests, the physician usually gives the patient topical applications of sulfonamide ointment or antibiotic eyedrops. When the specific bacteria are known, both systemic and topical therapy are used.

Prognosis

Acute bacterial conjunctivitis is almost always self-limited. If untreated, it lasts about two weeks; if properly treated, the course of the disease is milder, and it is usually cured in a few days. However, there are exceptions. Chronic bacterial conjunctivitis may not be self-limited and may become a problem to the subject.

ALLERGIC CONJUNCTIVITIS. Many air-borne agents can cause allergic conjunctivitis: pollen, animal dander, dust, cosmetics, and chemicals. Hay fever and upper respiratory infections are often accompanied by this type of conjunctivitis.

Findings

The subject has extreme itching and redness of the eyes, and tearing. If the nasal passages are involved, there will be nasal discharge and head congestion.

Treatment

Cold compresses help to relieve the itching. Topical corticosteroids and decongestant eyedrops give some relief. However, treatment is aimed at eliminating the cause of the condition, if the specific agent can be located. Otherwise, there are recurrences. Sometimes air conditioning and filtered air give dramatic relief.

Prognosis

Allergic conjunctivitis seldom threatens vision; also, both the symptoms and the severity of the attacks decrease as the subject becomes older.

Educational Implications

Any form of conjunctivitis should be taken seriously. Parents should be referred to an ophthalmologist or an eye clinic for appropriate care for their child.

Ophthalmia Neonatorum

At the present time ophthalmia neonatorum refers to a severe conjunctivitis occurring in the first ten days of an infant's life. There are at least three different types of organisms that may infect the baby's eyes during its passage through the mother's birth canal.

The time when the symptoms first appear is one way to identify the organism. The gonococcal disease appears two-three days after birth while another type may not appear for five to twelve days. The exact organism is identified by means of cultures and sensitivity tests.

Findings

Gonococcal conjunctivitis is often unilateral at first, but quickly becomes bilateral. The lids are swollen, and the conjunctiva becomes red and so swollen that it protrudes through the closed eyes. There is a purulent exudate.

Treatment

Weston (1979) advises that any case of acute, purulent conjunctivitis should be given immediate antibiotic therapy which may be adjusted after laboratory studies have identified the causative agent. Gonococcal conjunctivitis is treated by systemic penicillin, local antibiotics, and careful local hygienic measures.

The best treatment is prevention. The Crede 1 percent silver nitrate prophylaxis is effective for the prevention of gonorrheal ophthalmia. Scheie and Albert (1969) state that because of silver nitrate, this type of conjunctival infection now occurs in less than 0.03 percent of infants born in the United States today.

It is required by law that newborn infants have a 1 percent silver nitrate solution instilled into the eyes within minutes after birth. Prophylaxis for this type of gonorrhea was introduced by Crede in 1880. At present, in some places, the Crede treatment is being replaced by antibiotic administration; the advisability of this procedure is still controversial.

Prognosis

The cornea is involved less frequently if ophthalmia neonatorum is treated from the start. With proper treatment, the prognosis is generally favorable. If untreated, the disease remains acute for about five days, then slowly abates in four to six weeks. In such instances, the cornea is likely to become involved. This may result in a perforated cornea with loss of the eye.

Educational Implications

Children who have had ophthalmia neonatorum and enter the special education program have corneal scars as their main eye problem, scars which cannot be corrected with corneal transplants. Most of these children are in the program for the blind rather than for the partially seeing. The partially seeing make better use of their limited vision than would be expected from their visual acuity tests and eye examination reports. Such children should try low vision aids, such as magnifying glasses or special lenses, to determine if their vision can be further improved.

Listening to tapes and records, and typing from dictation, increase the amount of material these visually impaired children can assimilate.

Trachoma

Trachoma is now rare in the United States except among the Indians of the Southwest. However, the World Health Organization considers it the greatest single cause of progressive loss of sight. The disease has a world organization devoted to it, the International Organization Against Trachoma, and its own journal, *The International Review of Trachoma*. Furthermore, major trachoma studies are being conducted in all parts of the world, including the United States and Great Britain, where the disease itself is not a major problem.

Trachoma has existed for many centuries before Christ. Yet Thygeson (1967) states that until the introduction of sulfonamides in 1938, there had been no real progress in the treatment of the disease since the time of the Pharaohs. Fortunately trachoma has shown a marked tendency to disappear from countries whose standards of living have grown better and whose personal and family hygiene have improved. Nevertheless, in such areas as the Mediterranean basin, the Middle East, and the Orient, trachoma continues unchecked.

Trachoma is a chronic viral disease of the conjunctiva and cornea that spreads in the family as a result of close contact, as between mother and child or among siblings of preschool age.

The infection is hastened by poverty and poor hygiene, particularly in desert areas of the world where there is a lack of water. The disease causes visual loss and eye problems by forming scar tissue on both the conjunctiva and cornea.

Findings

The first symptoms of trachoma may resemble those of bacterial conjunctivitis: tearing, photophobia, pain, exudation, swelling, and redness of the bulbar conjunctiva. These are followed by follicles, keratitis, and the formation of a pannus. The disease is divided into four clinical stages:

1. There is thickening and swelling of the conjunctiva with the formation of small follicles in the upper tarsal conjunctiva.
2. Large follicles develop in the upper tarsus and become surrounded by inflammatory tissue. The upper part of the cornea usually becomes invaded by blood vessels from the limbus; this marks the onset of trachomatous pannus.
3. There is severe scarring and contraction. At first scarring is most evident in the conjunctiva of the upper lid. The lids become deformed and shorten. They may turn inward, causing the eyelashes to abrade the cornea, and result in scarring.
4. This stage represents healed trachoma since the disease is self-limited, and becomes arrested even without treatment. However, the sequelae remain.

When the conjunctival scarring is severe, it may close off the secretory ducts of the lacrimal glands, thus causing the eyes to become dry and the corneas opaque leading to visual loss. Other complications include ptosis, obstruction of the nasolacrimal ducts and dacryocystitis. Furthermore, because it is a chronic disease, trachoma often picks up secondary bacterial infections.

Treatment

In addition to sulfonamides, the trachoma virus is sensitive to tetracycline and streptomycin. Sulfonamides are usually given systemically and the antibiotic drugs topically.

Prognosis

Characteristically, trachoma is a chronic disease of long duration. In an ideal environment, however, about 20 percent of cases detected in any one year heal spontaneously; and when treatment is given early the prognosis is excellent. Unfortunately, however, because of unfavorable conditions and lack of treatment, some 20,000,000 people in the world today are blind from trachoma (Vaughan and Asbury, 1977, p. 66).

Educational Implications

Teachers of the visually impaired and others need to be aware of trachoma. It is possible that in their travels they themselves may become exposed to trachoma, or they may see or hear of persons with the disease. The teachers' knowledge of trachoma should enable them to know what procedures to follow.

REFERENCES

Becker, Bernard and Kolker, Allan. "Glaucoma." In *Vision and Its Disorders*. NINDB No. 4. Bethesda: U.S. Department of Health, Education, and Welfare, 1967, 87-113.

Gordon, Dan M. *Diseases of the Eye*. Summit: CIBA Pharmaceutical Company, 1962.

Martin-Doyle, J. L. C. *A Synopsis of Ophthalmology*. Bristol, England: John Wright & Sons, 1951.

Scheie, Harold G. and Albert, Daniel M. *Adler's Textbook of Ophthalmology*. 8th ed. Philadelphia: W. B. Saunders, 1969.

Scholz, Roy O. *Sight, A Handbook for Laymen*. Garden City: Doubleday, 1960.

Thygeson, P. "Problems in Trachoma Research." In *Vision and Its Disorders*. NINDB No. 4. Bethesda: U.S. Department of Health, Education and Welfare, 1967, 80-86.

Vaughan, Daniel and Asbury, Taylor. *General Ophthalmology*. 8th ed. Los Altos: Lange Medical Publications, 1977.

Weston, Horace L. Unpublished notes to the author, 10 p., 1979.

Chapter 5

DISEASES AND DEFECTS OF THE CORNEA, SCLERA, AND UVEAL TRACT, AND THEIR EDUCATIONAL IMPLICATIONS

THIS CHAPTER will discuss defects and diseases of parts of the eye that are actually concerned with vision.

THE CORNEA

Megalocornea

Megalocornea is an enlargement of the cornea that is almost always bilateral and is not progressive. This condition is usually inherited as a sex-linked recessive. It occurs almost exclusively in males.

Megalocornea may be accompanied by myopia, a deep anterior chamber, a large or dislocated lens, and some atrophy of iris tissue. There is no treatment, and if there are complications, the prognosis is not good. A dislocated lens may lead to glaucoma, and there may be cataracts in adult life.

Educational Implications

Usually there are some children with megalocornea in Detroit's program for the partially seeing. They are able to make satisfactory progress.

Keratoconus

Keratoconus or conical cornea is a cone-shaped protrusion of the center of the cornea caused by gradual thinning (Figure 13). It is a degenerative disease that is not evident until puberty and develops mainly in females. While the disease is almost always bilateral, one eye is frequently more affected than its fellow. Keratoconus is thought to be inherited through a recessive gene. It has been associated with other general diseases and also with certain eye diseases such as retinitis pigmentosa and aniridia.

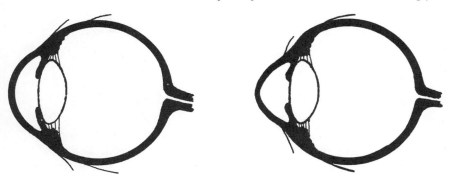

Figure 13. Comparison of normal cornea and keratoconus.

Findings

The earliest symptom is blurred vision, first in one eye, later in the other. Early in the course of the condition, the cornea looks normal, but slit lamp examination shows central thinning of the cornea and rupture of Descemet's membrane. Weston (1980) states that retinoscopic examination shows irregular astigmatism, which no lens can correct perfectly.

When the disease is well developed, the conical cornea may be seen by viewing the eye from the side, or by raising the upper lid and noticing the bulge as the subject looks down.

Treatment

In the early stages of keratoconus some ophthalmologists advise spectacles until the astigmatism becomes irregular, then contact lenses. Many ophthalmologists advise only contact lenses because they make the corneal surface smooth and thereby improve visual acuity. Actually, the contact lenses are not very satisfactory except in the early stages of keratoconus because they fit poorly and are uncomfortable. As the disease progresses and the corneas become thin, corneal transplants are recommended.

Prognosis

If the transplants are made before there is excessive corneal thinning, the prognosis is excellent. In fact, when corneal transplants are given these subjects, there may be a remarkable return of vision.

Educational Implications

The occasional child who has keratoconus as his primary condition is in the program for the partially seeing. This eye problem is generally recognized while the student is in junior high school. The special teacher may need to use his or her knowledge concerning the progressive nature of keratoconus to advise parents about the need for continuing medical care and counsel.

It may be irritating for the student to wear the prescribed contact lenses for long periods of time. Thus, the student should have his visual learning supplemented by auditory means, such as listening to recordings and tapes; also, his typing should include dictation. Such young persons need understanding and extra help with their studies since keratoconus develops at a difficult age.

Corneal Ulcers

Corneal ulcers may leave permanent opacities which seriously lower visual acuity. The complications which attend them may lead to loss of the eye.

> Scarring or perforation due to corneal ulceration is a major cause of blindness throughout the world. Most forms are amenable to therapy, but visual impairment can be avoided only if appropriate treatment is instituted promptly; in some cases this means within a matter of hours after onset (Vaughan and Asbury, 1977, p. 87).

There are many causes of corneal ulcers: bacteria, viruses, fungi, hypersensitivity reactions, avitaminosis A, exposure, and unknown causes. Pneumococcus is a common bacterial cause of corneal ulcers. Herpes simplex is the most frequent and troublesome of the viruses that cause ulcers. Other viral infections that may result in corneal ulcers are trachoma, herpes zoster, mumps, and measles. Fungal ulcers are more common in recent years than formerly. This increase parallels the topical use of antibiotics and steroids which enable fungi to grow in the cornea. The organisms enter the cornea following damage to the epithelium by trauma or inflammation. Many ulcers occur in subjects with nutritional deprivation and poor general health.

Corneal ulcers may be separated into central and marginal.

Central Corneal Ulcers

The central corneal ulcers result from a primary infection of the cornea by bacteria, viruses, or fungi. The normal corneal epithelium is a barrier against invasion. When ulceration does occur, it is usually the result of trauma which allows the entry of infection. The commonest central ulcer is that caused by pneumococcus bacteria (Streptococus pneumoniae). Its description follows.

The ulcer frequently starts at the margins of the cornea and progresses to the center. Because the lesion is snakelike in appearance, the ulcer is referred to as serpiginous. Hypopyon, a collection of pus in the anterior chamber, is commonly found. The pus is almost always sterile and is caused by the passage of bacterial toxins from the cornea into the anterior chamber.

Findings

The symptoms are severe. There is photophobia and pain in the eye. The pain is of two types: foreign body sensation and aching from the secondary iritis which always accompanies an acute ulcer.

Vision is blurred, especially if the lesion is in the central cornea. Tearing is usual. There is some swelling of the lids and conjunctival congestion. A grayish infiltration appears near the center of the cornea; this changes rapidly to an ulcer with sloughing margins. Surrounding the ulcer is a cloudy area; the rest of the cornea often is dull and gray. Unless treated, the ulcer spreads rapidly in both size and depth, destroying the cornea.

Treatment

Pneumococcus is sensitive to both sulfonamides and antibiotics, and local therapy is usually effective. Sedatives are given to ease pain and restlessness. Atropine may be used locally to control associated iritis. Rest and adequate diet are frequently considered important parts of the treatment.

If untreated, the cornea may be perforated. Corneal perforation is likely to destroy any hope of having vision in the eye and may possibly result in loss of the eyeball.

Prognosis

The extent of the loss of vision depends on the location and depth of the scar. Scar tissue which replaces the destroyed portions of the cornea usually fills in the gap so that the surface is level. However, scar tissue refracts the light rays irregularly. When Bowman's membrane is destroyed, it is never regenerated, and opacity remains. There is usually some degree of clearing eventually; this is more marked in younger subjects.

Occasionally a small dense scar covers the pupillary area during the healing of the ulcer. Vision may sometimes be improved through enlargement of the pupil by iridectomy. This operation is done after the healing is complete and there is no longer danger of stirring up infection.

Marginal Corneal Ulcers

Marginal ulcers are more common and usually more benign than those in the central cornea. They rarely result from a primary infection of the cornea. Instead, they result from toxic, metabolic, or metastatic processes often associated with conjunctival infection. There are two main groups of marginal ulcers: simple catarrhal and ring ulcers.

Simple catarrhal ulcers are seen on the periphery of the cornea. They are superficial, gray, and crescent-shaped. Usually the lesions occur as a complication of chronic conjunctivitis, but may occur secondary to conjunctival or systemic allergy. Catarrhal ulcers are benign and do not spread centrally. They frequently recur. Treatment is directed toward the conjunctivitis.

Ring ulcers extend around a portion or the whole of the corneal periphery. They are thought to be the result of a hypersensitivity reaction. The lesions usually are confined to the superficial stroma and rarely lead to perforation or extensive damage. The lesions tend, however, to become heavily vascularized. Treatment depends upon the symptoms.

Educational Implications

Corneal ulcers have become an infrequent cause of blindness and low vision in the Detroit Special Education Program. New medications as well as prompt medical aid and improved surgical procedures are responsible.

Teachers should be aware of the need for immediate medical attention for children who complain of persistent pain in the eye, photophobia, or blurred vision. Also, the teacher should check malnutrition and inadequate rest; both are contributing causes of corneal ulcers since they influence general health and resistance to infection. Magnifying glasses for close work may be helpful for children with corneal opacities.

Interstitial Keratitis

Interstitial keratitis is a severe keratitis in which blood vessels enter the stroma of the cornea. This disease is a late manifestation of congenital syphilis, but may be caused by tuberculosis or virus infections as well as by lesions of indefinite origin. It is considered a childhood disease since it usually appears between the ages of five and fifteen. The disease is more common in females than males.

Findings

The following findings concern syphilitic interstital keratitis. Hazy patches appear in the deep layers of the cornea or towards the center. If the patches start near the margin, they migrate toward the center; if at the center, others appear and fuse. Finally the whole cornea is lusterless and dull; later it becomes hazy.

Meanwhile vascularization has occurred. The vessels appear a dull reddish pink ("salmon patch") under the hazy cornea. If the subject does not receive treatment, this stage lasts from two to four months. The subject has pain, intense photophobia, lacrimation, and blepharospasm; these symptoms may be so severe that it is impossible for him to open his eyes. Vision may be reduced to hand movements.

After the interstitial keratitis has reached its height, the cornea clears slowly from the margin towards the center. As the cloudiness disappears, the vessels cease to carry blood, but remain permanently as fine lines in the cornea.

> The fine lines left by the collapse of the corneal blood vessels may be seen with a strong magnifying lens and suitable lighting, or the lines may be easily seen with a slit lamp. They interfere with vision much more than one might expect because they break up the orderly transmission of light rays (Weston, 1980, p. 2).

The corneal surface rarely becomes ulcerated. The uveal tract is always profoundly affected and iritis is present, sometimes severe uveitis. The keratitis is secondary; it merely masks the uveitis.

Treatment

The dominant treatment of syphilitic interstitial keratitis is penicillin in strong doses. Atropine is used to keep the ciliary body and iris at rest and to prevent the iris from adhering to the lens. In addition, topical corticosteroids are given. Dark glasses and a darkened room may be required for subjects with photophobia. Corneal transplants may be necessary for the corneal scarring.

Prognosis

The acute stage of interstitial keratitis may last from six weeks to several months. Clearing of the cornea takes many weeks or even months. The subject can expect little improvement in the cornea after eighteen months.

There may be relapses. The subject may need to be under treatment for a year.

Educational Implications

Most children and youth who develop this disease are now treated promptly and do not require special education. Those in the program for the partially seeing often do better close eye work, such as reading and writing, than would be expected from their vision and eye examination reports. In some instances, magnifying lenses enable the children and youth to see more clearly.

THE SCLERA

Staphyloma

Staphyloma consists of a bulge of thinned-out sclera that is lined with uveal tissue. This occurs as a result of either increased intraocular tension or thinning of the sclera. Staphylomas appear as dark blue, bulging areas in a particular part of the eyeball: anterior, equatorial, or posterior.

Anterior staphylomas usually occur over the ciliary body and are frequently associated with glaucoma. Posterior staphylomas may follow extreme myopia and are often associated with choroidal atrophy and retinal detachment. In fact, the staphylomas are usually the cause of the retinal detachment. The retina stretches little, if any, and cannot follow the expanding sclera.

Scleral tissue grafts have been used to correct staphylomas, but at the present time the prognosis is poor.

Episcleritis

Episcleritis is an inflammation of the episclera, the thin layer of vascular tissue between the sclera and conjunctiva. This is a fairly common, generally benign disease that is usually localized in the area between the limbus and the insertion of the rectus muscles. Episcleritis is often bilateral, occurs in young adults, and affects both sexes equally. The cause is not known, but hypersensitivity reactions are frequently responsible; also, certain systemic diseases such as syphilis, herpes zoster, and tuberculosis have been associated with episcleritis.

Findings

The most characteristic finding is the dull rose-color of the congestion. There is pain, photophobia, and some tearing. The conjunctiva and Tenon's capsule show swelling.

Treatment

Episcleritis lasts from one to two weeks. Topical corticosteroids reduce the inflammation in three or four days.

Prognosis

The condition has a tendency to recur and involve adjacent

areas. Although it may recur over a period of many years, it seldom leaves any residual ocular changes.

THE UVEAL TRACT

Aniridia

Aniridia is a congenital absence of the iris. However, some iris tissue is always present. This may consist of a root of the iris or a thin iris margin. Aniridia is almost always bilateral and is usually transmitted as a dominant characteristic.

Other defects of the eye are commonly associated with aniridia. The most frequent of these is congenital cataract; others include congenital glaucoma, corneal opacities, dislocated lens, incomplete development of the macula, photophobia, nystagmus, and strabismus. Scheie and Albert (1969) state that congenital glaucoma is present in more than half of the subjects with aniridia. Secondary glaucoma is likely to develop before adolescence when the lens is subluxated or otherwise dislocated.

Findings

The infant's eyes look large and black since the pupils are as large as the cornea. The amount of iris tissue in the two eyes may vary. The subject may have photophobia and nystagmus and vision no better than 20/200.

Treatment

The glaucoma associated with aniridia is difficult to control. If medical therapy is not effective, then surgery is necessary. Either goniotomy or trabeculotomy is the usual surgical procedure. When cataracts are present, it may be necessary to remove them in infancy or later in life, depending upon the extent and location of the opacity.

The low vision of subjects with aniridia may be due in part to the scattering of light at the margin of the lens. To correct this condition, contact lenses with pigmented peripheral portions and small, clear pupils are fitted to the subject. Such lenses may give him an improved image and reduced glare. Even when the subject does not obtain better vision with the lenses, the cosmetic results may be worthwhile.

Prognosis

The long-term prognosis for retaining good vision is poor.

Educational Implications

Detroit usually has some pupils with aniridia as their primary eye problem. Such children are able to function in the program for the partially seeing even though their binocular vision is seldom better than 20/200. Their low vision associated with nystagmus and photophobia makes school work difficult and discouraging. The children should have their desks in the part of the room where there are lower levels of illumination.

Since reading and writing are laborious for children with aniridia, they should have plenty of aural aids in doing their school work: records and tapes as well as large type books and materials, and typewriting from dictation. The children need more time to complete their assignments. Teachers should use some of the same procedures as for children who have albinism or nystagmus as their major eye problem. In addition, parents should be informed and guided in obtaining the services of an ophthalmologist or an eye clinic to determine if their child can profit from wearing special contact lenses.

Coloboma of the Iris

A coloboma is a congenital cleft or notch which is a developmental anomaly. It is caused by failure of two layers of tissue to close during fetal development, leaving a cleft between the two. The various types of colobomas are inherited as dominant traits. They are usually bilateral and may involve the iris, choroid, retina, optic nerve, and also the eyelids.

Typical colobomas of the iris are located in the lower part of the iris. The defect may be a small notch in the pupillary part of the iris or a severe defect in the uveal tissue. This condition is either unilateral or bilateral and occurs in both sexes.

Pigmented contact lenses with small, clear pupil areas have been used by children with severe types of iris colobomas.

Coloboma of the Choroid

Coloboma of the choroid is a congenital maldevelopment of

part of the choroid and retina. The coloboma is situated below the disc and may extend out to the ora serrata. It is usually bilateral and on ophthalmoscopic examination appears as a large white patch bordered with some pigment. The white appearance is caused by the absence of the choroid and retina in the area; only the sclera is visible. Sometimes the sclera is stretched and thinned over the area, and retinal blood vessels can be seen crossing it.

The visual field shows a scotoma which corresponds to the defect. Visual acuity is diminished and often strabismus and nystagmus are associated.

Albinism

Albinism is a disease affecting the metabolism of melanin, dark pigment. It is inherited as a recessive trait, and affects dark-skinned races more than light-skinned. The condition may involve the entire body (complete albinism), or only a part of the body (incomplete albinism). When incomplete albinism affects the eyes, their function may be normal or impaired. In complete ocular albinism, the iris, choroid, and retina are affected, and vision is greatly reduced.

Findings

Ocular signs of albinism are present at birth. The eyebrows and lashes are white, the conjunctivas are hyperemic, the irides either gray or red, and the pupils appear red. Ophthalmoscopically the fundus appears red and the macula is poorly developed. The absence of pigment in the choroid and retina makes the choroidal and retinal vessels stand out against the white sclera.

The subject has severe photophobia. His incompletely developed maculae make his vision defective; this results in an associated searching type of nystagmus. In addition, the subject may have a high error of refraction, usually myopia or myopic astigmatism.

Treatment

Treatment consists of corrective glasses, tinted to reduce the extreme amount of light entering the eyes. Contact lenses with painted irides and small, clear, or lightly tinted pupils may be recommended.

Educational Implications

At the present time 8.8 percent of the children in Detroit's program for the partially seeing have albinism. Their corrected visual acuity is about 20/200. This low vision, combined with photophobia, makes school work difficult. These children need special attention, assistance, and encouragement.

The teacher should be certain that children with albinism wear their prescribed glasses or contact lenses in order that they may obtain the best vision. They should be seated in the part of the room where there are lower levels of illumination. Children with albinism are often good students who are well organized and conscientious. However, they need more time (often twice as much as normally seeing children) to complete assignments, or they should have shortened assignments.

Typewriting increases their speed in completing assignments. Listening to tapes and records enables the children to assimilate more material in a shorter time. Closed circuit TV or special machines that enlarge and project on a screen the information they must read, are helpful.

Children with albinism of the hair and skin as well as of the eyes, occasionally develop psychological problems because of their appearance and the reaction of the others to it. The teacher should help these children gain competence in their academic work and should give them guidance in the development of social skills. Such special instruction and attention will increase their self-confidence and thereby help them to integrate with other children of the school.

Uveitis

Uveitis is a general term for the inflammatory disorders of the entire uveal tract. Although topographically separate, the iris, ciliary body, and choroid are closely related and form a continuous whole. Therefore, inflammations affecting the entire uveal tract will be considered together. Anterior uveitis is the preferred general term for iritis and iridocyclitis. Posterior uveitis is the preferred term for choroiditis and chorioretinitis.

(The retina is almost always secondarily infected in posterior uveitis.)

Among the many causes of inflammation of the uveal tract are infection, allergy, irritants, and toxic agents; also, uveitis is associated with noninfective systemic diseases, such as diabetes and diseases of the central nervous system. However, in most cases the cause of the uveitis is unknown. The inflammations are commonly unilateral and occur principally in the young and middle-age groups.

There are two broad types of uveitis: Nongranulomatous, the more common, and granulomatous. The nongranulomatous type is thought to be caused by hypersensitivity. It occurs mainly in the iris and ciliary body. Granulomatous uveitis is caused by the invasion of organisms, such as bacteria or fungi. This type may involve any part of the uveal tract, but is more common in the posterior area.

Findings

In the nongranulomatous type of uveitis, the onset is acute with marked pain, severe photophobia, and blurred vision. There is a flush surrounding the cornea caused by dilated limbal blood vessels. The pupil is small, but may be irregular if a posterior synechia is present. There is turbidity in the aqueous of the anterior chamber.

In granulomatous uveitis which commonly affects the posterior uveal tract, the onset is usually insidious with little or no pain, slight photophobia, but with marked blurring of vision. Only a slight flush surrounds the cornea and the pupil may be small or irregular. There is turbidity in the aqueous of the anterior chamber.

The retina is usually involved in granulomatous uveitis. Fresh lesions of the choroid and retina appear as yellowish white patches that are not seen clearly because of hazy vitreous. As these lesions heal, the vitreous clears and pigment is deposited at the edges of the patches. As a result of the healing process, considerable pigment is deposited. If the macula has not been affected, central vision remains good. A lesion in the pripheral retina may not be noticed by the subject.

Complications

Anterior uveitis may result in both anterior and posterior synechiae which impede the flow of aqueous, and thereby cause glaucoma. Interference with the lens metabolism may cause cataract; and retinal detachment may occur if there is traction on the retina by vitreous strands.

Treatment

Warm compresses and systemic analgesics are prescribed for pain in uveitis. Local steroid drops are used and the pupils are kept dilated with atropine. Dark glasses are required for the photophobia.

In granulomatous uveitis, the pupils are kept dilated if the inflammation is in the anterior segment of the eye. Dilation is very important to prevent an anterior synechia. Since a tentative diagnosis of the cause can often be made, specific therapy in the form of certain drugs is prescribed.

The complications associated with uveitis are also treated. When glaucoma is present, drugs, such as epinephrine, are used to inhibit the production of aqueous and reduce the intraocular pressure. If cataract results, it may be necessary to operate in order for the subject to have vision. If there is retinal detachment, it is treated even though the procedure is difficult in an eye with uveitis.

Prognosis

With treatment, nongranulomatous uveitis lasts from a few days to a few months. The prognosis is good and there is little or no interference with vision. However, recurrences are common.

Even with treatment, granulomatous uveitis may last from months to years. There may be remissions. The prognosis is fair to poor; frequently there is marked visual loss. Recurrences occur only occasionally. Without treatment, blindness ensues.

Educational Implications

There is always a small percentage of children in the Detroit program for the partially seeing whose low vision is a result of uveitis, both anterior and posterior. Such children have often had a long period of pain and frustration; they need much special attention and instruction.

Children and young persons whose acute uveitis does not permit them to enter school benefit from home instruction. Having a specially prepared teacher come into their home during school hours is a pleasant experience for these young persons and their parents. The special instructor teaches the children some of the required school subjects, thus giving them a goal to work toward. Some such young persons are able to accomplish half of their regular school program during a semester.

Sympathetic Ophthalmia (Sympathetic Uveitis)

Sympathetic ophthalmia is a granulomatous uveitis which can follow a perforating injury in the region of the ciliary body, iris, or lens; also, the disease may follow a retained foreign body. The injured (exciting) eye becomes inflamed first and the fellow (sympathizing) eye later; thus, the inflammation becomes bilateral. From the uveal tract the inflammation spreads to the optic nerve and its covering.

The cause of sympathetic ophthalmia is not known, but the disease is thought to be an allergy to the subject's own uveal pigment. If the injured eye does not begin to heal but remains red and swollen after a week or ten days, there is danger of the fellow (sympathizing) eye becoming inflamed even though it was not injured. Sympathetic ophthalmia may appear ten days to many years following the injury. The likelihood of this type of uveitis is greatest the first month after injury. From then on the chances decrease slowly but persist, in rare instances, for many years after the injury.

Sympathetic ophthalmia is less common than in former years for the following reasons: greater skill in the treatment of perforating wounds, stricter antiseptic precautions, and a greater tendency to remove an injured, sightless eye.

The incidence of sympathetic ophthalmia is not high, but it has devastating results. Children are considered particularly susceptible to the disease. They, more than adults, have accidents which involve penetrating wounds to the eye. Some of these wounds may go unnoticed or be neglected and thereby lead to sympathetic ophthalmia.

Findings

The subject complains of photophobia and blurring of vision. The eyes are red and there is tearing. If there has been a wound, the ophthalmologist looks for the scar where the injury occurred in the exciting eye. He uses a slit lamp to examine the anterior chambers of both eyes. Internal ocular signs of sympathetic ophthalmia include iritis or uveitis and hazy vitreous. The condition is diffuse rather than localized and is usually acute. The ophthalmologist considers it very important to recognize symptoms in the injured or exciting eye and he makes every effort to keep the inflammation from spreading to the sympathizing eye. Once the uveitis affects the sympathizing eye, prevention is impossible.

Treatment

The recommended treatment in a severely injured, sightless eye is enucleation to prevent sympathetic ophthalmia. When enucleation can be performed within ten days after injury, there is almost no chance that sympathetic ophthalmia will develop. When the inflammation has begun in the sympathizing eye, the usual treatment is local corticosteroids and atropine. In addition, systemic corticosteroids may be required. A child with sympathetic ophthalmia may need at least a year of intensive therapy.

Prognosis

Without treatment the disease progresses to total, bilateral blindness. With treatment there is likely to be some useful vision when the disease subsides.

Educational Implications

In recent years children with sympathetic ophthalmia are seldom found in the Detroit program for the visually impaired. However, special teachers need to be aware of the symptoms of this disease and its serious consequences.

REFERENCES

Andrews, Edson J. *Synopsis of Ophthalmology*. Tallahassee: The Florida State University, 1969.

Holt, L. Byerly (Ed.). *Pediatric Ophthalmology*. Philadelphia: Lea and Febiger, 1964.

Liebman, Sumner D. and Gellis, Sydney S. (Eds.). *The Pediatrician's Ophthalmology*. St. Louis: C. V. Mosby, 1966.

Scheie, Harold G. and Albert, Daniel M. *Adler's Textbook of Ophthalmology*. 8th ed. Philadelphia: W. B. Saunders, 1969.

Vaughan, Daniel and Asbury, Taylor. *General Ophthalmology*. 8th ed. Los Altos: Lange Medical Publications, 1977.

Weston, Horace L. Unpublished notes to the author, 25 p., 1980.

Chapter 6

DISEASES AND DEFECTS OF THE RETINA, OPTIC NERVE AND VISUAL CORTEX, LENS, AND VITREOUS, AND THEIR EDUCATIONAL IMPLICATIONS

THIS CHAPTER will conclude the discussion of defects and diseases of the eye and the related structures that are concerned with vision.

THE RETINA

Retinoblastoma

Retinoblastoma is rare, yet it is the most common intraocular tumor in childhood and the only malignancy that is known to be hereditary. The tumor arises from the retina itself and is fatal if untreated. Retinoblastoma attacks all races and both sexes. Involvement is bilateral in about 30 percent of the cases.

Some ophthalmologists consider the disease to be congenital. The average age at the time of diagnosis is thirteen months. Two-thirds of the cases are found before the end of the third year; occasionally cases are reported in later childhood.

The tumor arises spontaneously through a gene mutation or is inherited through a dominant gene that has high penetrance; that is, the gene is almost always able to produce its specific effect on the eye. The sporadic occurrence is more common, but the inherited variety seems to be increasing in frequency. This fact appears to indicate that more subjects are being cured of the disease. In the inherited or familial variety, the percentage of cases with bilateral involvement is significantly higher than in the sporadic.

Exhaustive studies have been made of the inheritance of both the sporadic and the inherited or familial varieties of retinoblastoma. A person who has survived the sporadic variety will have a 25 percent chance of producing affected offspring. An indi-

73

vidual who has been cured of the familial type will have a 50 percent risk that each of his children will be affected.

Findings

Retinoblastoma is usually unnoticed until one of the child's eyes shows a white pupillary reflex. Sometimes internal strabismus appears before the white reflex; this leads to earlier diagnosis. (Blind eyes of children often turn inward.) Otherwise, the tumor is seen in the early stages only when looked for in children having a hereditary background or when the fellow eye has been affected.

Retinoblastoma grows from the macular layers of the retina. Examination of the interior of the eye shows white, elevated retinal masses with indistinct borders. As the tumor enlarges and progresses, it may grow from the retina into the vitreous or into the choroid. If it grows into the choroid, it causes retinal detachment. In either situation the white pupillary reflex results. Further enlargement of the tumor is likely to lead to secondary glaucoma. The patient becomes photophobic and develops a steamy, enlarged cornea as in infantile glaucoma.

Degenerative changes in the eye with necrosis and calcification are frequent. The untreated tumor is slowgrowing and remains in the retina and vitreous for several months before it spreads to the brain by means of the optic nerve, or breaks through the sclera to invade the orbit. If this is allowed to occur, death usually results.

Treatment

Treatment consists of immediate enucleation of the involved eye when the condition is unilateral, with removal of as much of the optic nerve as possible. The fellow eye is examined every three or four months for three years following surgery, and at frequent intervals throughout childhood.

When retinoblastoma is bilateral, the eye with the more advanced lesion is enucleated. The fellow eye is treated with radiation or chemotherapy. However, if more than one-third of the retina is involved in the fellow eye, enucleation of this eye may be necessary in order to save the child's life (Scheie and Albert, 1969).

Treatment includes the examination and follow-up of the parents and all siblings of an affected child. In addition, the ophthalmologist is concerned with the eugenic counseling of parents, and their chances of producing more children with retinoblastoma.

Prognosis

Prognosis has improved greatly during recent years; this is mainly because cases are being uncovered at a much earlier stage than in the past. If the lesion is unilateral, diagnosed early, and treated promptly by enucleation, there is an 80 to 90 percent chance for survival. This high rate of cure decreases considerably when the tumor is bilateral.

It should be noted that at the present time there is a need for the perfection of other therapeutic methods for retinoblastoma. Such methods would include the preservation of the eye and its function in a larger percentage of subjects.

Educational Implications

At present there is a relatively high incidence of children with retinoblastoma in the Detroit program for the blind, 8.7 percent. These are usually children with the bilateral form of the disease; those with the unilateral form generally do not require special services.

Children with retinoblastoma have had painful and difficult years. Their vision is likely to be no more than light perception. Some have one artificial eye; others cannot wear a prosthesis because of the injury and scarring of their orbits in an effort to cure the disease. They should have all the aids and services available to supplement their school curriculum: the preschool teacher-counselor, orientation and mobility instruction, handcraft and music instruction given by special teachers, and reader service as they advance through school. Starting in the elementary grades they should learn to operate the typewriter with efficiency, and later with speed.

Surprisingly these children and young persons are frequently good students, some are superior. They are not apt to have emotional problems and are usually well liked by their classmates and teachers.

If a child with retinoblastoma complains of persistent pain in the eye, or if the teacher notices changes in the eye or surrounding structures, the child should be referred through his parents to an ophthalmologist.

Retrolental Fibroplasia

Retrolental fibroplasia, also known as the retinopathy of prematurity, is a bilateral disease of premature infants. The disease is considered to be a response of the infant's immature retinal vascular system to a high concentration of oxygen. The use of oxygen above that found in the normal atmosphere, 20 percent, includes a risk of inducing retrolental fibroplasia in premature infants.

The disease was unknown before 1940. At that time premature infants with irregular respiration were given high concentrations of oxygen. Retrolental fibroplasia was first described, named, and associated with Terry. In 1942 Terry reported a series of infants with the disease; all were premature and had gray-white membranes behind the lenses in both eyes. This condition was thought to be the result of prematurity.

In 1950 Gordon first suggested that the high concentration of oxygen given premature infants was in some way responsible for the disease. Kinsey of the Kresge Eye Institute, Detroit, was coordinator of a national study program which provided data on the relationship of oxygen to retrolental fibroplasia. In 1952 Campbell of Australia and Crose of England further confirmed the relationship of retrolental fibroplasia to the level and duration of oxygen therapy.

Scheie and Albert (1969, p. 149) state that the incidence of retrolental fibroplasia will increase with any one of three factors, each of which may act independently.

1. Oxygen concentration: the higher the concentration of oxygen, the greater the chance of the disease developing within a given period of time.
2. Duration of oxygen treatment: the longer the continuous oxygen treatment, the greater the risk of the disease developing.
3. Prematurity of the infant: if both of the above variables

are held constant, the smaller the infant, the greater the chance for the disease.

Findings

The eyes appear normal at birth. The disease has its onset during the first few days of life and may progress rapidly to blindness over a period of weeks. When blindness does occur, there is no hope of restoring sight.

With the use of a high concentration of oxygen, the retinal vessels first constrict, then become dilated and tortuous. Displacement of the retinal vessels may cause a migration of the macula to the temporal side. The retina swells and new blood vessels commence in the peripheral retina. These new vessels, along with connective tissue, may proliferate into the vitreous and cause retinal detachment by traction.

The retina becomes a fibrous mass which is seen as a dense membrane behind the lens, making the pupil appear white. The pupillary reflex is absent. The growth of the eye is usually arrested, and microphthalmos is likely to result. The anterior chamber is exceedingly shallow and anterior synechiae frequently cause secondary glaucoma. In fact, secondary glaucoma is present in approximately 30 percent of the severe cases of retrolental fibroplasia.

Other ocular findings associated with retrolental fibroplasia are corneal opacification, cataracts, and enophthalmos. Either of two types of strabismus may be present: esotropia when one eye is more damaged than the other, or exotropia when there is a temporal pull on the macula. Secondary nystagmus from decreased visual acuity is frequently present.

Regression

Once the activity has begun in retrolental fibroplasia, there is no way to predict at what stage it will stop, even though the infant is no longer receiving oxygen. However, spontaneous regression, which is a stabilization of activity within the eye, does occur, even in the early stages of the disease. The regression may be in one eye or both eyes. Myopia and strabismus are often found among those subjects who retain useful vision. This amounts to more than one-third of the infants. When there is scarring within the eye, the damage to vision is proportionate to the extent of the active stage of the disease. Another one-third or more of the infants do not have severe visual damage. On the other hand, it is estimated that approximately one quarter of the cases progress to the last stage of the disease which is complete blindness or merely light perception.

Treatment

There is no treatment for retrolental fibroplasia; the physician's major concern is prevention. Treatment of the secondary results of the disease may relieve symptoms or give improved vision. Refractive errors, such as myopia, are corrected with prescription glasses. When glaucoma is present, it usually occurs in eyes that are already blind. Miotics are prescribed. If there is some vision, surgery for the glaucoma may be necessary. Treatment of corneal scarring depends upon the location of the scar and the amount of retinal damage as well as the cosmetic appearance of the eye. Cataract removal may assist some subjects in obtaining better vision.

New cases of retrolental fibroplasia are now considered to be rare except for premature infants suffering from poor pulmonary function. Such infants have an increased survival rate when treated with high concentrations of oxygen. The physician monitors the infants to be certain they receive just enough oxygen to maintain an adequate blood oxygen level.

Prognosis

The prognosis is uncertain. Glaucoma, uveitis, retinal detachment or even phthisis bulbi may occur months or even years after the onset of retrolental fibroplasia.

Educational Implications

Only occasionally is a child with retrolental fibroplasia partially seeing; usually he is blind. At the present time 10.9 percent of the children and young persons in the Detroit program for the blind have retrolental fibroplasia as their primary eye problem. A number of these young persons have been in the program for many years. Michigan law permits visually handicapped persons to remain in certain special education programs until twenty-five years of age.

Children in classes for the blind with this disease usually have less residual vision than do those who are blind from certain other eye conditions. Those with retrolental fibroplasia may be totally without sight, have sheer light perception, or see only hand movements. Such children need many first-hand experiences and the aids and services available starting in preschool years.

The special teacher should be aware of the changes in the eyes of these children and persistent complaints about their eyes. Parents are then informed so that the children may be referred for medical eye care.

Retinal Detachment

The retina is firmly attached to the pigment epithelium layer at the disc and at the ora serrata, but between these points their surfaces are merely in apposition without any structural attachment. In retinal detachment the neural layer of the retina detaches or separates from the pigment epithelium. Scheie and Albert (1969, pp. 286-87) give three major mechanisms by which the retina can become detached.

1. Breaks, holes, or tears in the retina permit the escape of fluid from the vitreous into the subretinal space. In other instances, especially in younger subjects, the retina may be torn from its insertion at the ora serrata because of trauma or a congenital defect. Sudden trauma, such as a fall, or a penetrating injury may result in retinal holes.
2. Fibrous bands in the vitreous or vitreous shrinkage may detach the retina. Also, adhesions between the retina and vitreous, inflammatory exudates and hemmorrhages in the vitreous which organize and result in fibrous tissue formation, and new blood vessels in the retina which extend into the vitreous, are other causes of retinal detachment.
3. Subretinal fluid may accumulate from inflammation of the retina and choroid, from disturbances in the retinal

and choroidal circulation, and as a result of a systemic disease. These fluids and exudates may cause retinal detachment.

Most of the retina may become detached within a few hours, or it may take years. Scholz (1960) states that retinal detachment occurs more frequently in males than females.

Findings

The most common symptom of retinal detachment is the sudden appearance of many floating spots in the vision of one eye. Also, there may be recurrent flashes of light in a part of the field corresponding to the retinal tear or hole. The floating spots are caused by the entry of red blood cells or retinal pigment cells into the vitreous. The cells gain entrance by means of a retinal tear or hole. The retinal tear usually does not cause an immediate detachment; there is a progressive detachment with a consequent field loss. The subject may complain of a shadow or curtain coming up or down in front of his eye. However, the field loss often goes unnoticed because there is no pain and the subject retains good central vision until the macula is affected.

On ophthalmoscopic examination, the detached retina has lost its pink color and appears gray and opaque; it may tremble with every eye movement. If the detachment is well advanced, the separated area is bulged inward and thrown into folds.

The possibility of retinal detachment is greatly increased if the subject has had cataract extraction, is myopic, or has had an injury to the eye, either a contusion or a penetrating wound. Havener (1975, p. 391) states that almost half of all retinal detachment subjects have had cataract surgery. Detachment is more likely to occur if vitreous strands have run from the retina to the wound. Vitreous strands tend to contract in time, and, if they become firmly attached to the cataract wound, they may pull a hole or tear in the wound. The myopic eye is susceptible to retinal detachment because the eye has grown longer and larger since birth, thereby placing stretch on the retina which does not grow as rapidly as the outer coats of the eye. Such stretching makes the retina thinner and more liable to injury.

The subject's other eye must be examined since it often has

retinal holes or adhesions between the vitreous and retina which might lead to retinal detachment.

Treatment

Since a hole in the neural layer of the retina predisposes the eye to retinal detachment, surgical repair is necessary. The holes are usually in the peripheral retina and there may be multiple ones. The ophthalmologist makes a careful examination to be certain he locates all the holes or tears. The goal is to seal the holes and prevent others from developing. The holes or tears are sealed by three methods: freezing (cryotherapy), burning by light (photocoagulation), or burning by electricity (diathermy). These procedures irritate the choroid and pigment layer of the retina, inducing scar tissue formation that seals the holes.

Certain auxiliary procedures are used in retinal detachment operations.

1. The patient is put in a position that will help the retina to settle into place; for example, a detachment of the upper part of the retina is more able to settle if the patient remains lying down.
2. The fluid that lies between the two layers of the retina is drained at the time of surgery; this permits the two layers of the retina to come in contact again.
3. Implants of various types may be used to indent the sclera, choroid, and pigment layer of the retina towards the detached portion.

Prognosis

Ophthalmologists differ in their opinions as to the prognosis. Their estimates vary from 70 to 90 percent that retinal detachments can be repaired in one operation. If the operated retina remains in place after six months, it is not likely to become detached again.

Approximately 5 to 10 percent of detachments that are considered operable will continue to develop new holes or problems.

The fovea may suffer severe damage if separated for only a short time from its blood supply, the choriocapillaris. If involved in the detachment, the macula is usually damaged enough to preclude normal vision. If uninvolved, there may be normal vision after successful surgery.

The extrafoveal retina is better nourished by retinal blood vessels than is the fovea and thereby is able to withstand deterioration from detachment for a much longer time. Even after several months of detachment, the patient may have essentially normal extrafoveal vision if the retina is successfully reattached.

Educational Implications

Retinal detachment is an infrequent cause of blindness or very low vision in the Detroit special education program. Children and young persons with this condition have usually had a previous history of eye pathology such as degenerative myopia or aphakia. They are generally in the upper elementary or secondary grades and have become active physically in sports of various kinds.

Those with bilateral detachments naturally have a difficult time adjusting. At the beginning, the special teacher may concentrate on typing and listening skills, leaving Braille reading and writing until later. The young person is likely to be eager for orientation and mobility instruction, and he may participate in some of the many craft and music activities that are taught the visually impaired. Crafts, in addition to being an avenue of enjoyment, will increase the sensitivity of his fingers and thereby prepare him for learning Braille.

A child or young person in the program for the partially seeing may have a retinal detachment in only one eye. In such instances, the ophthalmologist is likely to instruct the teacher to restrict physical activities. For example, the young person may not be permitted to dive while swimming or to take part in contact sports, such as wrestling.

Macular Degeneration

The macular degenerations of children are commonly primary disorders and are hereditary. However, some are secondary to systemic diseases.

Two of the primary diseases will be discussed, Best's Vitelliform and Stargardt-Behr.

BEST'S VITELLIFORM DEGENERATION. This is a dominant disorder that is congenital or may have an onset as late as seven years of age. It is usually bilateral. Best's degeneration begins with cyst-like changes in the macula; the lesion becomes yellow-red in color. There are deposits in the pigment epithelium. Initially vision is good. Later the macula becomes pigmented and atrophic, causing central vision to be seriously reduced.

STARGARDT-BEHR DISEASE. This form of macular degeneration is usually recessive but may be dominant. It occurs between the ages of six and twenty. The disease begins with a rapid loss of vision, but ophthalmoscopic changes may not be seen. Within a year the macula begins to show pigment clumping. This may progress to a circular or oval area of degeneration. Peripheral vision is usually retained.

At present these hereditary macular degenerations are untreatable.

Retinitis Pigmentosa

Retinitis pigmentosa is a retinal pigment degeneration and not an inflammatory condition, as the name implies. In the disease the retinal rods are slowly destroyed; this is accompanied by a secondary atrophy of the remainder of the retina including the pigment epithelium. The etiology is unknown. Most frequently retinitis pigmentosa is a recessive trait, but it may be dominant or sex-linked. The onset of the disease is generally in the early teens. It is more common in males than females and is almost always bilateral.

Findings

The first symptom of retinitis pigmentosa occurs in early youth, or even in childhood, with night blindness. At the onset this symptom may have no physical findings. Then the retinal pigment epithelium degenerates and appears as black pigmented spots scattered throughout the midperiphery and especially distributed along the blood vessels. The process spreads both centrally and peripherally, the retinal arterioles become attenuated, and the disc atrophies, appearing pale and yellow. As the disease progresses the subject usually develops cataracts because the nutrition of the lens is disturbed; in addition, glaucoma and myopia are associated eye findings.

As time goes on, the fields continue to contract until only a tiny central area remains. The subject is unable to move about because he no longer has peripheral vision. Furthermore, his central vision may diminish slowly over the years.

When a person with retinitis pigmentosa reaches forty or fifty years of age, he may have only 3 to 5 degrees of central vision. In some instances, this is sufficient for him to be able to read for many years.

Treatment

At the present time there is no treatment for retinitis pigmentosa. Genetic counseling should be given the parents or the young adult in an effort to avert the propagation of this disease.

Educational Implications

The percentage of children with retinitis pigmentosa in the Detroit program for the blind is 6.5 percent, and is increasing. The incidence is 2.5 percent among the partially seeing.

Occasionally this condition appears in very young children who show head nodding in their effort to focus on a printed page, or as they do other near-point work. More often the disease shows itself when the student is in junior high school and goes from a sunny sports field into a dimly lighted locker room. He may be entirely disoriented. Others show their first symptoms when the days shorten and they must start for school before daylight.

These young partially seeing persons may be retarded in reading because of seeing words rather than phrases as they read.

When a student's central vision remains good so that he is able to read print instead of Braille, his greatest need is for orientation and mobility instruction. The instruction will enable the child or youth to go independently from one class to another within the school. Assistance with mobility will enable him to travel to and from school independently, and to travel in his neighborhood.

If his central vision is lost, it becomes necessary for the child or youth to learn Braille reading and writing. Most young persons are reluctant to learn Braille as long as they have central vision.

Typewriting becomes an important avenue of written communication and a quick way of doing some of the assignments. Special instruction in handicrafts and music provides avenues of participation and growth.

THE OPTIC NERVE AND VISUAL CORTEX

Coloboma

Colobomas of the optic nerve exist separately or within large choroidal colobomas. When separate, the coloboma may be of little significance and appear as a crescent at the lower margin of the disc. More commonly the coloboma is about four times the size of the disc, and blood vessels emerge around its edge. A coloboma may involve the entire disc or only the lower part. A blind spot corresponding to the area of the colobomatous defect is usually present. In the more severe optic nerve colobomas, the vision is usually grossly defective. There is no treatment.

Optic Atrophy

Optic atrophy is a degeneration of the optic nerve in any part of its course. Optic atrophy may be caused by a lesion in any one of the following places: in the retina, at the optic disc, or anywhere in the optic nerve or optic tract between the globe and the lateral geniculate body.

Weston (1980) lists the following causes of this degenerative condition:

Occlusion of the central artery or vein
Neuritis of the optic nerve or tract due to inflammations, as in multiple sclerosis, and toxins, such as methyl alcohol
Consecutive atrophy which is secondary to retinal disease
Increased intraocular pressure, as in glaucoma
Trauma to the optic nerve or tract by injury, tumor, abscess, or aneurysm
Metabolic diseases such as diabetes
Hereditary diseases
Increased intracranial pressure from any cause.

In addition, optic atrophy may be genetically determined.

This occurs in both a recessive and dominant form. The recessive form is present at birth or within two years and is a more severe form. The dominant form has its onset during childhood, and progresses little thereafter. In this form the child characteristically has blind spots in the field of vision and thereby a loss of visual acuity.

Findings

Loss of vision is the main symptom. The loss may be in visual acuity, in the visual field, or a combination of both. Ophthalmoscopically, optic atrophy is characterized by pallor of the optic disc. The pallor of the disc and loss of pupillary reaction are generally proportionate to the loss of vision.

In complete optic atrophy, the pupils are dilated and fixed, and the patient is blind. When the atrophy is partial, the pupil reactions are sluggish and vision is subnormal. The fields are usually contracted and have abnormal blind spots.

Treatment

Treatment is limited to that of the condition causing the atrophy. As already noted, pressure against the optic nerve may cause visual loss. However, if the pressure can be relieved before nerve fiber death, vision may be regained.

Usually the underlying cause of optic atrophy cannot be treated effectively.

Prognosis

The prognosis is generally not favorable. There may be a slow but progressive deterioration of vision. However, some cases in which the etiological condition can be stopped may remain stationary as partial atrophy. Examples are an injury with the trauma having ceased and intracranial pressure being removed.

Educational Implications

At the present time optic atrophy accounts for 15.2 percent of children in the Detroit program for the blind. It is one of the three primary causes of blindness. Fewer children in the program for the partially seeing have this disease; at present, only 1.7 percent.

It is often difficult to determine the visual status of children with optic atrophy. They may or may not have some central vision. When central vision is fairly good, the child may read small chalkboard writing more easily than large.

Some children may have such poor peripheral vision that they are unable to find nearby objects without using their hands to search. Obviously, they require orientation and mobility instruction.

Those children who have some vision frequently derive much benefit from low vision aids, such as magnifiers and telescopic lenses.

Cortical Blindness

Cortical blindness is caused by a lesion in the occipital lobe. Such lesions may result from destruction of cortical tissue as in injury, tumor, or degeneration. If both lobes are extensively injured, there can be total blindness.

This condition is suspected if the pupils respond normally to light and the fundi show no changes, but all other signs indicate that the child is blind for educational purposes.

At the present time 4.4 percent of the children in the Detroit program for the blind have cortical blindness. Such children may have good visual acuity in a small field, but the peripheral field is greatly reduced, making it difficult for them to move about. The children require orientation and mobility instruction, and the other aids and services to blind children, starting as soon as the condition is diagnosed.

When the child is old enough, his visual fields may be plotted to determine their size. Any refractive errors are corrected with glasses. These children need much understanding and encouragement as they learn to cope with their visual loss.

THE LENS

Dislocated Lens (Ectopia Lentis)

A dislocated or displaced lens results from some defect in the zonule, such as atrophy, rupture, stretching, or imperfect development. When the lens is partially separated from the zonules, it is subluxated; when completely separated from zonular and vitreous attachments, it is luxated. Three types of subluxated lenses will be discussed: congenital, spontaneous and traumatic.

CONGENITAL FORMS. In congenital forms the lens displacement is commonly upward and nasally. This anomaly is usually bilateral and symmetrical in the two eyes. The lenses frequently remain clear, but may develop cataracts.

If the lens is displaced so much laterally that the edge or margin crosses the pupil, the subject has uniocular diplopia. The lens margin is very astigmatic. Through the phakic portion of the pupil, the eye is myopic and very astigmatic; through the aphakic portion, it is highly hyperopic.

A dislocated lens may be one component of a generalized disturbance of growth, such as in Marfan's syndrome (arachnodactyly or spider fingers) and Marchesani's syndrome. Marfan's syndrome, the more common, is a disease of connective tissue which is passed on as a dominant characteristic that affects both sexes equally. The most striking feature of this syndrome is arachnodactyly, an increased length of the long bones, particularly of the hands and feet. It is estimated that 40 percent of the patients with this disease have eye anomalies, including displaced lenses. Scheie and Albert (1969, p. 23) state that Marfan's syndrome accounts for 70 percent of the congenitally displaced lenses.

Marchesani's syndrome is related to Marfan's. Persons with this condition are short and have stubby fingers and toes. Several eye anomalies, including ectopia lentis and glaucoma, are characteristic.

SPONTANEOUS DISLOCATION. Spontaneous dislocations that are subluxated may, as a result of complications, become luxated. Luxated lenses also occur in eyes with buphthalmos, staphylomas, or high degrees of myopia. In such diseases the enlargement or lengthening of the eyeball causes too great a strain on the zonules.

TRAUMATIC DISPLACEMENT. Traumatic displacement may occur following a blow to the eye. After such an injury, the eye is usually soft with a deep anterior chamber. If the blow is not severe, the eye recovers, with the lens returning to its regular position and the anterior chamber slowly becoming normal.

In any of the three types of subluxated lenses, the zonules may become ruptured, causing luxation. If the lens enters the anterior chamber, it may occlude the pupil area, thereby preventing aqueous flow. This leads to secondary glaucoma. However, the lens may remain in its normal position because of adhesion to the vitreous. In such instances, the lens floats in the anterior part of the vitreous causing the iris to become tremulous and shake with movements of the eye.

Findings

Displaced lenses may have some of the following symptoms: blurred vision, a change of refraction, interference with accommodation, monocular diplopia, a tremulous iris, and a red eye.

A displaced lens may frequently be seen through the pupil, especially if it has developed a cataract. When the lens is completely displaced into the vitreous, it can be seen with the ophthalmoscope.

Treatment

Lens displacements result in unusual refractive errors which necessitate careful testing for corrective glasses. The phakic portion of the pupil has extreme astigmatism and must be corrected before the aphakic portion. Continuous, regular use of mydriatics may be needed to furnish sufficient pupillary space. The lens may sometimes be removed to furnish an unobstructed pupil.

In total dislocation, secondary glaucoma is almost certain to develop and requires lens removal even though much risk is involved.

Prognosis

The prognosis for a dislocated lens is cautious. When the dislocation is partial and the lens remains clear, the visual prognosis is good. If the lens becomes cataractous or enters the anterior chamber, poor vision is likely to result.

Educational Implications

Children with dislocated lenses have sufficient vision to function in a program for the partially seeing. At the present time such children make up 1.7 percent of those in the program.

Reading and close eye work are difficult and laborious for the children. They need relief from periods of close eye work by such methods as doing part of their writing at the chalkboard, typing from dictation, and listening to some of their lesson material on tapes or records.

Specially fitted lenses and other low vision aids may benefit the children. Closed circuit television or machines which project an enlarged image of a book or written material on a screen are helpful.

Cataract

A cataract is any opacity or clouding of the lens. The opacity results from change in the physiochemical state of the lens proteins. The opacity may vary from a few spots to almost the entire lens. Among the causes of cataract in children are the following:

Heredity
Intrauterine infections, including rubella
Chromosomal aberrations, such as in Down's syndrome
Prematurity
Drugs, such as systemic steroids
Ocular diseases, such as glaucoma and uveitis which cause
  secondary cataract
Trauma
Inborn metabolic disturbances, such as diabetes mellitus
Systemic disorders, such as Marfan's syndrome.

Three types of cataracts will be discussed: congenital, traumatic, and galactosemia.

Congenital Cataract

Congenital cataracts may occur at any time during the embryonic formation of the lens. While most such cataracts are inherited as a dominant trait, others result from reactions to intrauterine infections or influences. They are mainly bilateral, but most are not dense enough to blur the vision notably and are not progressive. Others progress slowly and may not require surgery until the child is approximately fifteen years of age. The severity and rate of progression in each eye may vary.

Only those congenital cataracts that cause a significant loss of vision will be considered here.

Findings

The one symptom of cataract is impaired vision. It is usually the mother who notices that the infant does not see well during the first few months.

When the cataract is total, the pupil appears white. Slit lamp examination shows the density of the cataract, and may enable the ophthalmologist to tell the approximate time of its development.

The ophthalmologist considers the possibility of cataract if the child has strabismus, lowered visual acuity, a family history of the disease, and other ocular abnormalities and systemic defects.

Treatment

At present the only treatment for cataract is surgery. Surgery is done with caution for the patient who has congenital cataracts. If the cataracts are bilateral and dense so that the retinae are not clearly visible, the lens is extracted in one eye at approximately six months of age. The purpose of this early surgery is to permit the development of vision and prevent nystagmus. If surgery on the first eye is successful, the cataract can be removed from the second eye two or three months later. If not successful, surgery is delayed one or two years until the eye is larger and there is less risk of complications.

When the patient has cataracts resulting from rubella, surgery is delayed, at least until the age of two. One reason for the delay is that the live rubella virus is present in the eye, especially within the lens itself, for many months after birth. The virus may be released at the time of the operation and cause uveitis. Another reason for the delay in surgery is that rubella cataract may be associated with other ocular abnormalities. The most common of these is microphthalmos; others are opaque corneas, glaucoma, and iridocyclitis. The ophthalmologist wishes to be certain that it is the cataract, and not another eye anomaly, that is causing the blindness or low vision.

After surgery, the child must be fitted with corrective glasses or contact lenses to compensate for the loss of his lens.

Prognosis

The prognosis for congenital cataract is guarded. Patients with senile cataract have a better visual prognosis. Vaughan and Asbury (1977, p. 140) estimate that no more than 70 percent of operations for congenital cataracts result in significantly and permanently increased visual acuity. Rubella cataract has the worst prognosis for good vision.

The operation for congenital cataract is complicated and anomalies of the retina and optic nerve associated with the cataract may decrease the amount of useful vision. In addition, months or years following the operation, vitreous strands may develop which upon contraction cause retinal detachment. Fortunately, such retinal detachments may be treated by surgery in many of the patients.

The most favorable prognosis is for the child with normal intelligence who has bilateral cataracts, but no other ocular abnormality. A unilateral cataract is generally associated with a deep amblyopia which surgery does not correct. When the child is older such a cataract may be removed for cosmetic reasons.

A child with dense cataracts in both eyes may never learn to fixate objects properly due to the failure of macular vision to develop. Nystagmus may result from this lack of fixation ability even though the cataracts were successfully removed.

Traumatic Cataract

A traumatic cataract may result from a blunt injury such as a blow to the eye. Such an opacity may clear up in days or weeks, but more frequently is permanent. Unless the opacity is dense, there is little impairment of vision. If a penetrating injury is slight, such as inflicted by a needle or thorn, it may seal over before significant damage is done, but the injured eye is likely to become cataractous before its fellow eye even years later. When a penetrating injury or a foreign body such as a BB shot or a stone, pierces the capsule of the lens, aqueous and vitreous may enter the lens structure. The eye may become red and painful. This causes opacification of the lens within a short time, a few hours or a few days. The wound at the entrance to the eye may be large enough to permit aqueous and vitreous to escape. The eye then becomes soft and may develop complications such as infections, uveitis, and retinal detachment.

Findings

The patient with traumatic cataract complains of blurred vision. The eye becomes red.

Treatment and Prognosis

Most concussional lens opacities do not progress and often have little effect on vision. Thus, they do not require special treatment. If the capsule is ruptured and the lens swelling causes secondary glaucoma, the lens material is washed out in order to reduce tension and improve vision. When a foreign body enters the eye, damaging the lens, it is extracted along with the lens material, and the wound repaired. Treatment which may consist of antibiotics and corticosteroids is given to prevent the development of infection.

In children and young persons under twenty years of age, the lens material in a traumatic cataract will often absorb during a period of months without an operation. When a membrane remains and interferes with vision, an incision is made into the lens capsule to break it up so that it may absorb more readily.

Galactosemia Cataract

Galactosemia is a congenital disease in which the infant is unable to metabolize galactose. The disease is manifest soon after birth and is frequently associated with the development of bilateral cataracts in early life.

These cataracts are reversible providing that milk and milk products are eliminated from the diet in the early stages of galactosemia.

Educational Implications

At the present time cataract is the major cause of blindness and an important cause of low vision in Detroit's special education program. Cataract accounts for 21.8 percent of the blind children and 9.5 percent of the partially seeing. These statistics show the seriousness of this eye disease. The larger percentage of children are blind and do not use their eyes as the main avenue of learning. Starting in preschool years, they will need all the aid and services available to the blind.

If the aphakic child is able to function as a sighted person, he may have corrected visual acuity of approximately 20/70. Aphakic children, since their eyes no longer have the power of accommodation, nearly always need bifocal lenses in their glasses. If they wear contact lenses, they will require glasses for near vision.

The special teacher will be alert to changes in vision and complaints of these children. It is usually at the secondary school level that young persons with cataracts develop added complications. The special teacher, even more than the parents, may understand the necessity of having the child referred to an ophthalmologist or an eye clinic.

If a partially seeing child has a central lens opacity, he will have trouble in bright illumination when the pupil of the eye is contracted. His vision is better at lower levels of light. Thus, his desk should be located in the area of the room where there is less light. As the child becomes older, his pupils decrease in size. Occasionally drugs for dilating the pupils are prescribed so that the young person can see around the cataract.

Children with a central lens opacity, especially those in beginning reading, may read more easily when looking through a slot made in black construction paper placed on the printed matter. The slot exposes two or three lines of print.

When the opacities are in the periphery of the lens, the child's visual acuity is better in good light. His desk should be placed in a well-lighted part of the room. However, a light that is too bright reflects the rays against the cataract and causes glare.

VITREOUS

Vitreous Degeneration

Vitreous degeneration, liquefaction, and shrinkage may occur with pathologic myopia, injury, or inflammation. Injuries and inflammations may result in hemorrhage and inflammatory exudates in the vitreous cavity. These lesions may be followed by the formation of membranes, vitreoretinal adhesions, and large liquid pockets. Months or even years later, such conditions may lead to retinal detachment.

In some children, especially those with a family history of retinal detachment, there may be a specific kind of vitreoretinal degeneration. This condition is characterized by areas of retinal thinning with overlying pockets of vitreous liquefaction. These lesions may lead to retinal breaks or holes.

Fluidity is caused by coagulation of the proteins of the vitreous so that the gel structure is disrupted. Opacities usually indicate that the vitreous is fluid.

There is no treatment for fluidity. When an operation is necessary, and vitreous escapes, it can be replaced by an intraocular fluid. The volume of the intraocular fluid will be maintained by the normal formation of aqueous.

REFERENCES

Havener, William H. *Synposis of Ophthalmology.* 4th ed. St. Louis: C. V. Mosby, 1975.

Harley, Robison D. (Ed.). *Pediatric Ophthalmology.* Philadelphia: W. B. Saunders, 1975.

Ophthalmic Staff of Hospital for Sick Children, Toronto. *The Eye in Childhood.* Chicago: Yearbook Medical Publishers, 1967.

Pagon, Roberta A. "The Role of Genetic Counseling in the Prevention of Blindness." *Sightsaving Review* 1979-80, 49, 157-65.

Scheie, Harold G. and Albert, Daniel M. *Adler's Textbook of Ophthalmology.* 8th ed. Philadelphia: W. B. Saunders, 1969.

Scholz, Roy O. *Sight, A Handbook for Laymen.* Garden City: Doubleday, 1960.

Vaughan, Daniel and Asbury, Taylor. *General Ophthalmology.* 8th ed. Los Altos: Lange Medical Publications, 1977.

Weston, Horace L. Unpublished notes to the author, 25 p., 1980.

Chapter 7

OPTICS AND ERRORS OF REFRACTION

THE FIRST PART of this chapter will be concerned with optics, the science that deals with light. This science forms the basis of the diagnosis and correction of optical difficulties of the eye. The second part of the chapter will discuss these optical difficulties which are known as errors of refraction, and how they are "corrected" or neutralized by optical means.

OPTICS

Light is a form of radiant energy which gives objects visibility. Light travels from its source in straight lines or rays. When the light source is close, such as an electric lamp 2 feet away, the rays are divergent when they reach the eye. When the light source is 20 feet (6 meters) or more away, the divergence is so slight that for practical purposes the rays are considered parallel.

When rays of light pass obliquely from one transparent medium into another of different optical density, they are bent or deflected. This bending is known as refraction.

Prisms

A prism is a solid, wedge-shaped piece of glass or plastic that changes the direction of light rays passing through it; the deviation is at both the surface of entrance and the surface of exit (Figure 14). Entering rays are deviated toward the base, the thicker part, but continue the same relationship (parallel, converging, or diverging) while passing through and after emerging from the prism. A prism diopter (Δ) is used to express the strength of a prism. A degree (°), another unit of measurement of a prism, equals about 2Δ.

Prisms are used (1) to determine if an eye has a tendency to turn, (2) to decide how much a deviating eye turns, (3) to neutralize the effects of extraocular muscle insufficiency, and (4) to use in therapy exercises for weak extra-ocular muscles.

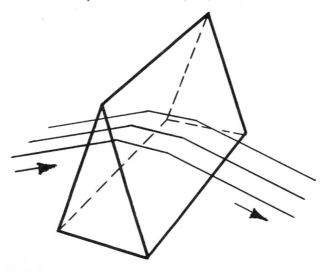

Figure 14. Prism refracting light rays toward the base.

The position of a prism when placed in an eyeglass is indicated by the direction of its base. "Base in" means that the base or thick part is toward the nose. The base may be in (◁), out (▷), up (∇) or down (Δ).

Many (probably most) doctors prescribe as ⊃ 5Δ in and 2Δ up instead of calculating the axis angle (Weston, 1980, p. 12).

Spherical Lenses

A lens is a piece of glass or plastic with one or both surfaces curved; it bends or refracts light rays toward or away from its principal axis, the imaginary line through its center perpendicular to its surface. There are two basic types of lenses, spherical and cylindrical, and combinations of these. Spherical lenses have at least one surface which is the segment of a sphere (one may be plano or flat), and refract light rays in all meridians or planes. There are two kinds of spherical lenses, convex and concave.

In optical illustrations, lenses and prisms are usually diagrammed in cross section to avoid the confusion of three dimensional drawings (Weston, 1980, p. 12).

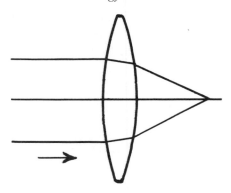

Figure 15. Convex lens converging light rays.

CONVEX LENSES. Convex lenses, in cross-section, may be considered as two prisms of continually changing angle or power with bases together at the center and with outward curved surfaces. Such lenses are thicker in the center than at the edge.* Parallel rays of light passing through a convex lens will be converged and brought to a focus behind the lens (Figure 15). Convex lenses are known as converging, magnifying, positive, or plus lenses, and are designated by the sign +.

CONCAVE LENSES. Concave lenses may similarly be considered as two prisms of continually changing power with the apexes together at the center and with incurved surfaces. Such lenses are thinner at the center than at the edge. Parallel rays of light passing through a concave lens will be diverged and thus will not come to a focus behind the lens (Figure 16). If these rays are projected backward, they form a virtual or imaginary image on the same side as the object. Concave lenses are known as diverging, reducing, negative, or minus lenses and are designated by the sign −.

Cylindrical Lenses

A cylindrical lens or cylinder is a segment of a cylinder parallel to its axis. Cylindrical lenses are either convex or concave. Light passing through a cylinder in the plane of its axis is not refracted.

---

* The toric construction (forward bulging) of spectacle lenses makes smaller thickness differences difficult to detect, especially in sphero cylinders.

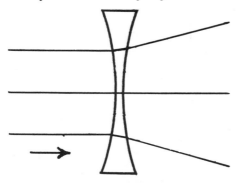

Figure 16. Concave lens diverging light rays.

However, when light passes through in a plane other than that of the axis, the rays become either convergent or divergent, depending upon whether the cylinder is convex or concave (Figure 17). The amount of convergence or divergence depends upon the angle between the plane of the rays and that of the cylinder axis. Refraction is greatest in the plane at right angles to the axis. It is necessary to indicate the angle at which the cylinder is placed before the eye.

Numbering Lenses

Weston (1980) explains the numbering of lenses. The strength of a lens refers to its refractive power and the unit of measurement by which it is expressed is the diopter (D), the power which will bring parallel light rays to a focus at 1 meter. The stronger the refractive power of a lens, the closer is its focal point. To facilitate optical calculations of combinations of lenses, the diopter is defined as the reciprocal of the focal length in meters: $D = 1/m$. Thus, a 2.00 D lens will have a focal length of ½ meter and a 4.00 D lens, ¼ meter. For fractional powers ⅛ diopter steps are used, expressed as decimals, but with the third decimal place omitted, but understood, i.e. 0.12 D, 0.25 D, 0.37 D, 0.50 D, 0.62 D, 0.75 D, and 0.87 D. To avoid errors the full two decimal places should always be expressed, even if zeros. Likewise, a figure is always placed before the decimal point, even if zero, i.e. 0.25 and 3.00.

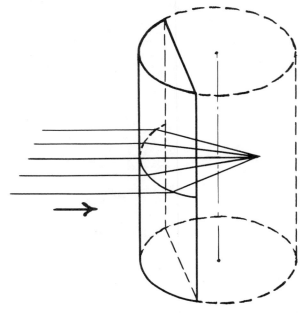

Figure 17. Convex cylindrical lens showing focus in plane at right angles to the axis.

The dioptric system allows direct algebraic additions of powers. Convex or converging lenses are designated as plus because of their power to produce a focus, and concave lenses are designated minus because they have only virtual or imaginary focusing power, which, however, is useful in reducing or compensating for excessive converging power, i.e. a combination of + 1.00 D, + 0.25 D = 1.25 D and + 2.50 D − 1.75 D = + 0.75 D.

Recognizing Different Lenses*

Those who teach visually impaired children should know how to recognize different kinds of spherical and cylindrical lenses. In moving a spherical lens across a page 3 or 4 inches above the

* The student should be helped to recognize lenses by actually handling and examining them. Lenses may be obtained from spectacles no longer being used or from an optical firm. It is best to first introduce spherical lenses of high refractive power, such as a convex lens used for cataract correction, or a concave lens used to correct severe myopia. Next the student should examine spherical lenses of lower refractive power, then cylindrical lenses.

surface, the print will appear to move rapidly if the lens is strong, slowly if the lens is weak. If the print seems to move in the opposite direction to the movement of the lens, and the print appears enlarged, the lens is convex or $+$. If the print seems to move in the same direction as the lens, and the print appears smaller, the lens is concave or $-$.

Examining the lens itself will be an additional means of identifying it. The convex lens is thicker in the middle while the concave lens is thinner in the middle. Most spherical lenses are combined with cylindrical lenses since almost everyone has some astigmatism.

To identify a cylindrical lens, a horizontal or vertical line, such as on the edge of a door or chalkboard, several feet from the observer is located. The lens is then rotated a few degrees in front of the eye while looking at the horizontal or vertical line. The straight line will appear to twist or turn in the opposite direction if the cylinder is convex; in the same direction if the cylinder is concave.

REFRACTION*

The eye may be considered an optical instrument. Rays of light entering the eye pass through the cornea, the aqueous, the lens, and the vitreous to focus on the retina. Light rays are first converged at the cornea and then by the lens, the former having 2½ times the effect of the latter. In the normal eye which is observing distant objects, the incoming light rays are essentially parallel and will focus on the retina. Objects at distances which are nearer than 20 feet are observed with diverging rays requiring additional focusing power which is accomplished by accommodation in which the lens of the eye changes curvature as required. The cornea takes no part in accommodation.

Eyes in which incoming parallel rays do not focus on the retina when accommodation is at rest are said to have refractive errors; these will be discussed later. The procedure of measuring the refractive power of the eye and its errors has come to be known simply as performing "refraction."

---

* Much of the material on refraction was written by Dr. Horace L. Weston, May, 1980.

Changes in Accommodation

Accommodation is present from the earliest age at which it can be measured, approximately 6 months, at which time it is strong, until old age when it is weak. The loss in accommodative power is due to hardening of the lens substance, making it more resistant to changes in shape, and to the ciliary muscle losing some of its tone. The decline is at a rather constant rate until the mid-forties when it accelerates slightly, but slows abruptly at about age fifty, there being little accommodation remaining to be lost.

In childhood and youth there is so much reserve power of accommodation that the decline is not noticed; in the twenties there is some trouble with seeing very fine near work; and by the mid-forties there is difficulty with reading ordinary print. When there is significant inability to focus on near objects, the condition is called presbyopia.

Presbyopia ("old sight") may be accompanied by headache and fatigue when near visual work is attempted. A convex spherical lens of suitable strength placed before the eye or added to one's distance correction, if glasses are needed, will enable the individual to read at the ordinary distance. This lens may be separate in reading glasses, bifocals, or trifocals. Younger individuals with low visual acuity may also be helped with the use of additional magnification for reading.

Emmetropia

Emmetropia ("sight in proper measure") is the condition in which an eye has no refractive error. It requires that all of the measurements of the eye be exactly correct in order that incoming parallel light rays will be focused on the retina without the assistance of accommodation (Figure 18). The noted authority, Duke-Elder (1969, p. 58) has stated, "emmetropia may be optically normal, but it is no more biologically normal than would be the universal attainment of a uniform height of 5 feet 6 inches." Because of variations in physical growth, emmetropia is seldom found.

Ametropia

Ametropia ("away from" emmetropia) is the condition in which the eye has a refractive error. The three main types of errors are hyperopia, myopia, and astigmatism.

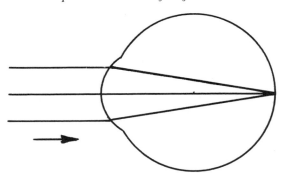

Figure 18. Focus in emmetropia.

Anisometropia is not in itself a refractive error but may be included here. Anisometropia is the condition or state in which the refractive errors of the two eyes differ significantly in type or degree. The unequal magnification of anisometropic corrections may cause sufficient differences in image size, known as aniseikonia, to produce eyestrain symptoms.

Eyes with refractive errors frequently have associated symptoms and other findings, especially in children. Among these are rubbing the eyes, blinking, frowning, closing the eyes, tilting the head, photophobia, reddened conjunctiva, and tearing. Blepharitis may be a symptom of ametropia as are red and swollen eyelids. Headaches, dizziness, and nausea occasionally result from refractive errors.

Hyperopia (Hypermetropia)
(Farsightedness)

In hyperopia parallel rays of light are brought to a focus behind the retina (Figure 19a). Hyperopia is commonly caused by shortness of the eyeball, but occasionally results from weakness of the refractive power of the cornea or lens. Hyperopia may be associated with underdevelopment of the eye and other congenital defects.

When the hyperopic eye is small or underdeveloped, the diameter of the cornea is likely to be reduced and considerable astigmatism is often present. In addition, the anterior chamber is shallow; this is partly due to the lens being of normal size. This condition predisposes the eye to glaucoma.

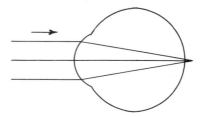

Figure 19a. Hyperopia, uncorrected.

Findings

Hyperopia, unless extreme or astigmatic, does not usually interfere with vision in children because of their good reserve of accommodation. In low amounts, there may be no symptom, but moderate or high errors are likely to cause difficulty chiefly due to the need for an excessive amount of accommodation and the lack of balance between accommodation and convergence.

Children with hyperopia are likely to have eyestrain or asthenopia. The eyes ache and burn so that blinking movements are more frequent than normal. There is tearing. A history may reveal that the child tires easily and has headaches. In addition, he finds it difficult to read or do other near point work.

In severe hyperopia, the eyes may not develop good visual acuity, attaining only 20/40 or 20/50 or less instead of 20/20 or better at seven years of age. Distant vision may be kept only by accommodative effort, and near vision is blurred even with excessive accommodation. Such a hyperopic child will become disinterested in reading and near work because he cannot obtain a clear image. This may lead to his having a short attention span.

Hyperopes have a smaller retinal image than do myopes. The average hyperope does not have quite as high corrected visual acuity as does the myope even with equal health of the retina.

Most hyperopes have some astigmatism. They have well-developed ciliary muscles. In young children hyperopia is a predisposing cause of convergent strabismus (Chapter 8). The presence of heterophoria increases the tendency to headache.

A cycloplegic drug should be used before refracting the eyes, and an annual eye examination is advised.

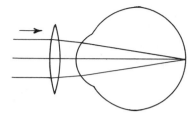

Figure 19b. Hyperopia, corrected with convex lens.

Treatment

Hyperopia is corrected with a convex or plus spherical lens of sufficient strength to add the necessary additional convergence to incoming rays of light so that they will come to a focus on the retina (Figure 19b). Correction of moderate degrees of hyperopia for children without symptom or heterophoria may not be necessary. In fact, heterophoria without symptom is seldom corrected in children, or even in adults. There is a great individual variation in tolerance to heterophoria.

Prognosis

Hyperopia decreases gradually until about age twenty-five. The prognosis is good if children who are given corrective lenses wear them. Corrective lenses may relieve eyestrain and prevent strabismus, in addition to giving better visual acuity.

Educational Implications

At the present time 3.8 percent of the children in the Detroit program for the visually impaired have hyperopia as their primary eye difficulty. These children do not adjust readily to near vision activities. They may tire easily when using their eyes at close range. Short periods of concentration on close work and interesting material help them. The pupils should make much use of the typewriter, especially in typing from dictation and in composing. They may respond best to material on an overhead projector or to a film or film strip projected on a screen.

A hyperope who has gone without his glasses for some time may have considerable trouble adjusting to them. The child is likely to complain that the glasses do not help. His higher interpretive visual centers have not been receiving the proper stimulation. The child must learn to see more clearly; this process takes time and constant wearing of his glasses.

Myopia (Nearsightedness)

In myopia parallel rays of light are brought to a focus in front of the retina (Figure 20a). Myopia is usually caused by an increase in the axial length of the eyeball but may result from an excessive amount of refractive power in the cornea or lens. Generally myopia first becomes evident during the early years of school and continues to progress until after the teen years. It is particularly likely to manifest itself at the age of puberty. Myopia is strongly hereditary.

Two kinds of myopia are recognized, simple and degenerative. Simple myopia is considered to be solely a refractive error due to the excessive growth of the length of the eyeball. Degenerative or malignant myopia is not identified by the strength of the correcting glasses, but by ophthalmoscopic examination of the retina and choroid. Degenerative myopia is much less common than simple. It has a higher incidence in females than males.

Myopia may be associated with other anomalies of the eye, such as albinism. An end result of retrolental fibroplasia may be high degrees of myopia with poor visual acuity in both eyes.

Findings

The one symptom of all myopia is the inability to see clearly in the distance. Parents are likely to notice that the child holds any

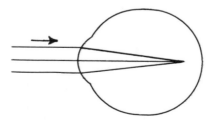

Figure 20a. Myopia, uncorrected.

object he wishes to examine close to his eyes. The teacher may observe that the child cannot see the numbers on the clockface, bends over to work at his desk, or holds his reading book close to his eyes. However, the child does not complain about reading since there is usually no strain on accommodation.

The myopic child may frown in an effort to see in the distance; this can result in a headache. Some children squint their eyes so that there is only a tiny hole through which to look. This procedure eliminates the peripheral light rays, leaving only the central rays which give a clearer image.

Eyestrain is a much less prominent symptom in myopia than in hyperopia, but it does exist due to several reasons and may be manifest as tired eyes, headaches, and blepharitis. The myope does not have the strain of excessive accommodation for near vision that the hyperope has. However, he is much more likely to have eye muscle strain from exophoria and the resulting disproportion between the efforts of accommodation and convergence. Eyestrain in myopia may be more marked if there is associated astigmatism or anisometropia.

The typical myope has a deep anterior chamber. The increased length of the eye occasionally causes it to appear more prominent than normal. In degenerative myopia there is likely to be poor vision even with optical correction, and the subject is likely to have photophobia and see black spots floating before his eyes.

The subject with degenerative myopia may have the following changes within his eyes: (1) a temporal crescent, the myopic crescent, which is an area where the choroid and retina pull away from the edge of the disc and expose the sclera; (2) a chorioretinal deterioration of the macula which appears as a heavily pigmented area; (3) a localized stretched sclera which generally forms a posterior staphyloma and thus increases the myopia; and (4) vitreous detachment and degeneration.

Treatment

Myopia is corrected with a concave or minus lens which will diverge incoming light rays in sufficient degree to neutralize the excessive convergence and focus the rays on the retina (Figure

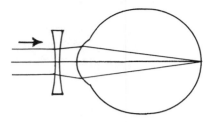

Figure 20b. Myopia, corrected with concave lens.

20b). Some ophthalmologists do not recommend corrective lenses for children who have mild degrees of myopia, − 1.00 D or − 1.50 D.

> It is true that in younger children myopia of − 1.00 D or less, or even − 1.50 D may not need correction. My own opinion was to consider the uncorrected vision and what was needed to see the chalkboard work in school. A − 1.00 D error usually limits uncorrected vision to about 20/40; I consider this the minimum for classroom work (Weston, 1980, p. 16).

The degenerative myope is corrected with concave lenses as long as they can increase the visual acuity. At the present time there is no other satisfactory treatment for this condition. The progressive nature of myopia makes it necessary for children and young persons to have an annual eye examination.

Prognosis

The prognosis for simple myopia is good; many persons maintain normal or near normal vision with proper corrective glasses providing they do not have additional complications such as nystagmus or severe astigmatism. The prognosis for degenerative myopia is poor for the following reasons: thinning of the choroid leads to the loss of retinal functioning in the involved area, changes in the macula greatly reduce central vision, and opacities from vitreous degeneration reduce vision. The retinal degeneration and stretching make the retina liable to tears and detachment. Cataract and secondary glaucoma may be associated with degenerative myopia.

Because of the gravity of the prognosis of degenerative

myopia in later life, the following statement was made by an ophthalmologist:

> Consideration should also be given to the hereditary propogation of the disease; at least, two high myopes with pronounced degenerative changes in the fundi should not have children. (Miller, 1978, p. 88).

Educational Implications

Myopia is the primary visual difficulty of children in the Detroit special program who are partially seeing. At the present time 48.3 percent of these children and young persons have this condition. Some have myopia of the degenerative type. Others have additional anomalies such as severe astigmatism, nystagmus, or albinism.

Myopic children who do not have other anomalies, may have a tendency to read for long periods of time because it is easy for them. Myopes who have otherwise healthy eyes are not affected by the reading they do. However, the children frequently have a tendency to lean over their work. They should be expected to use desks with adjustable tops or reading stands, to read under good lighting conditions, and to have good posture.

Typewriting is an important part of the curriculum for myopic children. As soon as they have learned the keyboard, they should start doing some of their assignments on the typewriter. Also, they may type from dictation, compose, and copy passages for practice.

Some myopic children need to be encouraged and helped to be more outgoing. They should take an active part in the oral phase of the reading program. Their interests should be broadened to include outdoor sports and activities. Good health, adequate diet, and outdoor exercise should be emphasized.

Children with degenerative myopia have delicate eyes that are liable to retinal detachment. They are advised to avoid active and contact sports such as football, wrestling, and boxing. Their ophthalmologist may recommend that they do not dive when swimming.

Glasses usually give the myopic child much better visual acuity; therefore, he is not likely to complain about wearing them.

Nevertheless, teachers and parents should be aware of a statement made by a world-famous ophthalmologist.

> Children should wear their distance correction constantly — not particularly in the interests of their eyes, but in the interests of their mental development — for children with even low degrees of uncorrected myopia cannot be expected to take a normal interest in their surroundings since they cannot see distant objects as clearly as their fellows. Their mental horizon is constricted, they tend to become unduly introspective, and they are thrown more and more into finding their interest in reading and near work (Duke-Elder, 1970, pp. 85-86).

Astigmatism

In astigmatism ("a" without; "stigma," point) there is a variation in refractive power along different meridians of the eye. Each meridian will focus parallel rays of light at a different place or spot, so that the image is a line, oval, or circle, but not a point. Astigmatism is commonly caused by the cornea being more curved in one direction than another, but occasionally it results from changes in the lens. As in other refractive errors, heredity is an important factor, and nearly all astigmatism is congenital. Astigmatism may be regular or irregular.

REGULAR ASTIGMATISM. In regular astigmatism the varying refractive powers in different meridians can be placed into two principal meridians at right angles to each other. In astigmatism with the rule, the vertical meridian (of the cornea) has the greater curvature. Children and young persons commonly have astigmatism with the rule. In astigmatism against the rule, the horizontal meridian (of the cornea) has the greater curvature. The lens of the eye tends to have astigmatism against the rule and this may become evident in later life due to flattening of the cornea with age.

The pattern which light rays take after traversing the cornea and lens is similar in all astigmatic eyes, but five types are described, according to where the foci of the stronger and weaker meridians lie in relation to the retina.

1. Simple hyperopic astigmatism: one meridian is emmetropic and the other is hyperopic (Figure 21).
2. Simple myopic astigmatism: one meridian is emmetropic and the other is myopic (Figure 22).

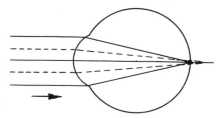

Figure 21. Simple hyperopic astigmatism.

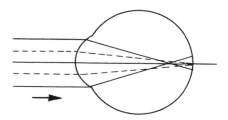

Figure 22. Simple myopic astigmatism.

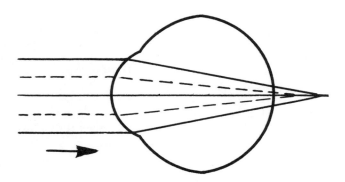

Figure 23. Compound hyperopic astigmatism.

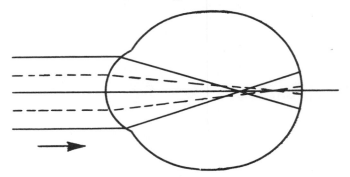

Figure 24. Compound myopic astigmatism.

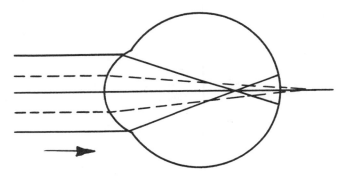

Figure 25. Mixed astigmatism.

3. Compound hyperopic astigmatism: both meridians are hyperopic. The astigmatism is combined with hyperopia (Figure 23).
4. Compound myopic astigmatism: both meridians are myopic. The astigmatism is combined with myopia (Figure 24).
5. Mixed astigmatism: one meridian is myopic and the other hyperopic (Figure 25).

IRREGULAR ASTIGMATISM. In irregular astigmatism there is a difference in refraction not only in varying meridians, but also in different parts of the same meridian. Injuries to the cornea which result in scarring, irregularities of the lens, or keratoconus are the usual causes of irregular astigmatism.

The following material will concern *regular* astigmatism unless stated otherwise.

Findings

Eyestrain and blurred vision are common symptoms of astigmatism. While some children may adjust to astigmatism without symptoms, others have indefinable symptoms such as headache, irritability, fatigue, or nervousness. Young children may become discouraged quickly and cry easily.

In lower grades of astigmatism, there is always diminished acuteness of vision, both near and distant, depending upon the degree and type. However, the images are seen well enough to stimulate an almost constant effort at accommodation. This is likely to result in headache and pain after using the eyes for close work or after prolonged attention at a distance, such as at a theater or when riding in a car.

In higher grades of astigmatism the images are so blurred that there may be no attempt to improve them by accommodation. The subject accepts a reduction in vision.

Astigmatism is suspected when vision cannot be improved with spherical lenses even though there is no apparent eye disease or abnormality. The astigmatic dial is a common method for determining astigmatism. The dial is formed of radiating lines numbered like the face of a clock. When placed before the dial, the subject is unable to see all the lines with equal distinctness. The line seen most distinctly and the line seen least distinctly indicate the axes of the two principal meridians. Each eye should be examined separately.

Treatment

Astigmatism is corrected by prescribing cylindric or spherocylindric glasses which correct the error. The curve of the correcting cylinder corresponds to the ametropic meridian. The axis of the cylinder which may vary from 0 to 180 degrees, is fixed in the glasses at right angles to the ametropic meridian. The axis, or angle, at which the cylinder is placed may be at any angle between horizontal and vertical according to the angle of the ametropic meridian.

It is not always possible to obtain normal vision with full correction, but the visual acuity is likely to improve after the glasses have been worn for a time. Glasses should be worn constantly if the subject is to obtain relief from his symptoms.

Irregular astigmatism may be improved by contact lenses which tend to make the cornea more spherical, as in the early stages of keratoconus.

Children and young persons with either regular or irregular astigmatism should have annual eye examinations with a cycloplegic drug.

Prognosis

Most astigmatism stays fairly constant.

Educational Implications

Whether the astigmatism is basically myopic or hyperopic, it is not a primary cause of eye difficulties in the Detroit Program for the Visually Impaired. After determining whether the astigmatism is hyperopic or myopic, the teacher will use many of the procedures for children with either of these refractive errors.

It should be stressed that children who have astigmatism should wear their glasses. The glasses should be kept straight in order to correct the error.

Less Common Types of Ametropia

ANISOMETROPIA. Refractive errors tend to be quite symmetrical so that a comparable amount of hyperopia or myopia will be found in each eye. Occasionally a subject has a considerable difference in the amount of refractive error in each eye; this is anisometropia.

The eye with the higher refractive error tends to have poorer visual acuity. If anisometropia is discovered during the first three or four years of life, glasses are prescribed to develop good vision in the poorer eye. A young child may tolerate unequal correction in the two eyes whereas an older child cannot. After six or seven years of age, there is little chance of improving vision in the poorer eye when the anisometropia is more than mild. As a result, the child will commonly use one eye exclusively and suppress the vision of the other eye.

ANISEIKONIA. Aniseikonia is a difference in the size of the retinal image in each eye. In anisometropia the unequal magnification from the unequal corrections for each eye will produce retinal images of unequal size which may be difficult or impossible to fuse. When each eye has nearly equal corrected visual acuity the child may use one eye, then the other, but not both together. This is one cause of uniocular or "alternating" vision. Contact lenses can be·used by some to diminish the optical defects of glasses. For others, it may be necessary to undercorrect the more ametropic eye.

Methods of Refraction

When an ophthalmologist examines children's eyes for refractive errors, a cycloplegic drug is used. This drug temporarily paralyzes accommodation in order to measure the refractive error of the eye when it is at rest; the state which glasses will, hopefully, create. Also, the drug dilates the pupil, enabling the doctor to more easily examine the interior of the eye.

In examining the interior or fundus of the eye for possible disease, an instrument, the ophthalmoscope, is used. An ophthalmoscope has a selection of various lens powers which enable the examiner to focus at different levels within the eye and to compensate for refractive errors of the eye. With careful use an approximate estimate of the refractive error of the eye may also be determined.

During the fundus examination the disc, macula, and major blood vessels are observed. The purpose is to detect possible anomalies and diseases that may or may not be associated with the refractive error.

The refraction portion of the examination may be either objective or subjective. The objective determination of refractive errors is made with the retinoscope or one of the recently developed more sophisticated optical devices. Its use involves the observation of the movement of focused light emerging from the subject's eye. These movements have patterns that are characteristic of hyperopia, myopia, and astigmatism. With the aid of the retinoscope, the proper lenses to correct the refractive error can be determined. By using this instrument, the refractive error of an infant can be measured accurately.

The subjective method of refraction involves asking the subject to distinguish between the effects of lenses on the visibility of letters or symbols on a chart. This method is used for adults and for children old enough to recognize the letters or symbols. The subjective method may be used to check results obtained by the objective method.

Prescription of Lenses

The purpose of prescriptive lenses is to improve visual acuity and to relieve symptoms caused by the refractive error. These prescriptive lenses may be either spectacles or contact lenses. Spectacles or glasses are generally worn by children.

Most low-visioned children in programs for the visually impaired require glasses. Some cannot increase their vision with glasses and therefore do not wear them. Children in the general school population who have only slight refractive errors and no symptoms may not need glasses. Children with anisemotropia frequently require glasses to prevent the development of amblyopia in the poorer eye. In addition, corrective glasses may check a tendency to muscle imbalance and thereby prevent strabismus.

There are two kinds of contact lenses, hard and soft. Unless otherwise indicated, this discussion will refer to the hard lenses. Contact lenses continue to increase in popularity. They provide good optical quality, and a better field of vision without peripheral distortion, than do glasses. Contact lenses may usually be worn all day after being properly fitted. Ophthalmologists recommend them for severe myopia or hyperopia, for unilateral aphakia in order to retain binocular vision, for bilateral aphakia, and for keratoconus. Contact lenses are frequently worn during athletic activities. However, the main reason for wearing them is still cosmetic.

There are some disadvantages of contact lenses. The subject needs considerable training in inserting and removing them. It is not easy to obtain corneal tolerance, and there are occasionally corneal abrasions and erosions. Injury of the cornea followed by infection can result from careless use of contact lenses. Because of the possible hazards, the lenses should be fitted under medical supervision.

The newer soft contact lenses offer longer wearing time, but less sharpness of vision. Many subjects readily adjust to them. However, the soft lenses have a potential for absorbing harmful fluids. At the present time many ophthalmologists consider hard contact lenses to be superior to the soft. The hard lenses are more durable, easier to insert and remove, easier to clean, and less expensive.

As yet there are no definite rules about contact lenses for children. Some children with high refractive errors can wear the lenses successfully at five or six years of age; most cannot. An important criteria for use of the lenses is motivation on the part of the subject. Children are usually not motivated for contact lens wear before the ages of thirteen to fifteen. At that time they may be eager to have them, but many cannot wear them after they have been fitted.

Reading Prescriptions

The professional eye specialist may not always specify the name of the refractive error on his examination report. The special teacher will recognize the refractive error by reading the prescription for the corrective glasses. In fact, reading the prescription will give the teacher a better understanding of the condition.

A prescription for lenses is written by placing the sign (+ for convex, − for concave) before the strength in diopters. This is followed by the designation of the sphere (S or sph) or cylinder (cyl) with its axis in degrees (°).

> The angle at which the axis of a cylinder is placed is indicated in degrees away from the horizontal in a counter-clockwise direction as viewed facing the wearer. The 0-180° line is horizontal, 45° to upper left and lower right, 90° vertical, and 135° to upper right and lower left. To avoid confusion, the 180° designation is always used for horizontal — although the same, 0° might be misunderstood (Weston, 1980, p. 18).

When a sphere and a cylinder are combined, a symbol, ⌒ , meaning combined with, is used. The abbreviation O.D. (for oculus dexter, right eye), and O.S. (oculus sinister, left eye) are used to designate the eye for which the lens is prescribed. The abbreviation O.U. (oculus unitas, both eyes) indicates that both eyes have the same prescription for lenses.

This is an example of a hypothetical prescription:

O.D. +2.50 D S ⊃ +3.00 D Cyl ax 95.

This means, for the right eye, a plus 2.50 diopter spherical lens is combined with a plus 3.00 diopter cylindrical lens. Frequently only the bare essentials are included. Thus, the above prescription is written:

O.D. +2.50 +3.00 x 95.

A value without an axis marking is a sphere; with an axis indicator (x), a cylinder.

The following are examples of other prescriptions:

O.D. +2.75 sph
  Right eye, hyperopia
O.U. −4.25 S
  Both eyes, myopia
O.S. +3.00 x 100
  Left eye, simple hyperopic astigmatism
O.D. −4.00 cyl ax 175
O.S. −3.75 −4.25 cyl ax 180
  Right eye, simple myopic astigmatism
  Left eye, compound myopic astigmatism
O.U. +3.25 +3.75 x 85°
  Both eyes, compound hyperopic astigmatism
O.D. −5.00
O.S. −5.25 −4.50 x 175
  Right eye, myopia
  Left eye, compound myopic astigmatism
O.U. +1.75 sph −2.25 x 180
  Both eyes, mixed astigmatism. In mixed astigmatism, the cylinder is larger than the sphere and opposite in sign.
O.S. +2.50 +2.75 x 25 ⊃ 2 Δ up.
  Left eye, compound hyperopic astigmatism with a prism correction for hyperphoria.
O.D. +12.00 +1.00 x 90 add +3.00
  Right eye, very high compound hyperopic astigmatism as in cataract glasses, with bifocal addition.

REFERENCES

Brent, H. P. Contact Lenses for Children. In Ophthalmologic Staff of Hospital for Sick Children, Toronto, *The Eye in Childhood*. Chicago: Yearbook Medical Publishers, 1967, 482-88.

Duke-Elder, Stewart. *Parsons' Diseases of the Eye*. 15th ed. London, England: J. and A. Churchill, 1970.

Duke-Elder, Stewart. *The Practice of Refraction*. 8th ed. St. Louis: C. V. Mosby, 1969.

Miller, Stephen, J. H. *Parsons' Diseases of the Eye*. 16th ed. New York: Churchill Livingstone, 1978.

Morgan, A. L. and Arstikaitis, Maria. Refraction. In Ophthalmologic Staff of Hospital for Sick Children, Toronto, *The Eye in Childhood*. Chicago: Yearbook Medical Publishers, 1967, 19-27.

Refractive Anomalies of the Eye. NINDB Monograph No. 5. Bethesda: U.S. Department of Health, Education, and Welfare, 1967.

Spaeth, Philip G. and Heyman, Louis S. Corneal and Scleral Contact Lenses in Children. In Robison D. Harley (Ed.), *Pediatric Ophthalmology*. Philadelphia: W. B. Saunders, 1975, 753-60.

Vail, Derrick. *The Truth About Your Eyes*. 2nd ed. New York: Farrar, Straus and Cudahy, 1959.

Weston, Horace L. Unpublished notes to the author, 25 p., 1980.

Chapter 8

STRABISMUS

BINOCULAR VISION means the ability to see with two eyes, but the term is commonly used to designate the simultaneous viewing of the same field with both eyes. In normal binocular vision an image of the object being looked at falls on the fovea of each eye producing impulses which are carried from the retinae, along the visual pathways, to the occipital cortex where they are combined in the perception of a single image. This merging of the two separately received images into one is called fusion.

Each eye has its own field of vision (monocular field) which differs from that of its fellow eye in being wider on the temporal side. For the most part, the monocular fields overlap producing a central, binocular field, but each eye has an outer area of vision not seen by the other (Figure 26). This outer area helps to locate objects toward which the more discriminating, central binocular vision may be directed.

Figures 27 and 28 illustrate binocular vision. In Figure 28, the man is seen with central vision, the dog with peripheral. Since the dog is about 20 degrees from fixation, it would be seen with visual acuity of only 0.1. The image of the dog would be rather blurred.

When the eyes are placed so that the image falls on the fovea of one eye but not on the other, the second eye is deviating or squinting, and strabismus is present. Approximately 3 percent of all children have this condition.

The infant is likely to show occasional deviations of eye movements during the first six months. However, if he shows constant strabismus even before six months, he should be referred to an ophthalmologist. The ophthalmologist may be able to begin early treatment; if not, he may at least make periodic examinations and find the general cause of the strabismus.

It cannot be emphasized enough that the visual system, including good visual acuity, fusion or blending of cerebral images into one, and

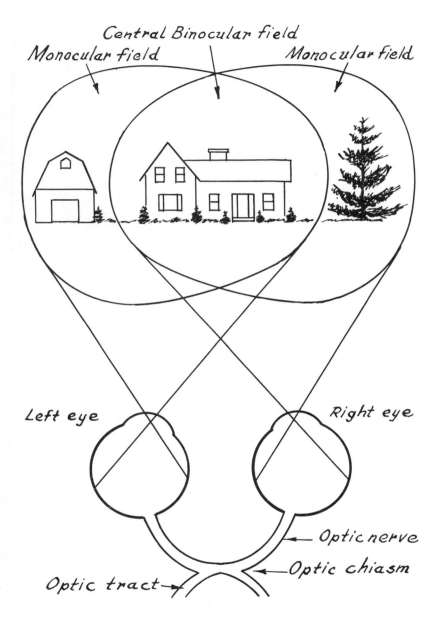

Figure 26. The visual field

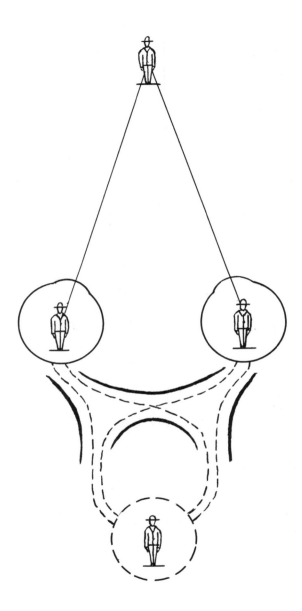

Figure 27. Binocular vision.

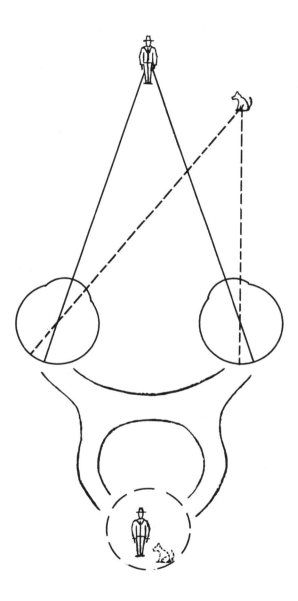

Figure 28. Binocular vision, central and peripheral

proper motor (muscle) coordination must follow a normal course during the first 6 years of life. The eyes must be used together for as much of this period as is possible. Although the potential for normal binocular cooperation is innate, bad sensory habits established in strabismic patients during the first 6 years of visual development may be so profound as to be practically irreversible (Jampolsky, 1964, p. 211).

After six or seven years of age, the components of vision are likely to be set. Prolonged treatment may improve visual acuity, but normal binocular vision may not always be obtained.

CAUSES OF STRABISMUS

Among the causes of strabismus are anomalies in the structure of the eyes or in the extraocular muscles, defects or deviations of innervation, or defects in the center of fusion in the brain.

Anomalies of Structure

Since every movement of the globe involves the action of its six extraocular muscles, a defect in size or attachment of any one of the muscles can inhibit smooth binocular coordination and rotation of the eye. Refractive errors, particularly high hyperopia and refractive differences between the eyes (anisometropia), are important causes of strabismus. Any lesion interfering with vision such as opacities of cornea or lens, retinal scars and defects, or even tumors may cause ocular misalignment.

Deviations of Innervation

The third cranial nerve, the oculomotor, controls not only four of the six extraocular muscles, but also the functions of accommodation and convergence. These closely associated reflexes result in excessive convergence when there is excessive accommodation, as in uncorrected hyperopia. As a result, fusion may break down and the eyes turn in. This usually occurs at 2 or 3 years of age when the child becomes interested in clearly focusing on objects and toys near him.

The fourth and sixth cranial nerves, the trochlear and abducens, supply the other extraocular muscles, the lateral rectus, and superior oblique.

Defects of Fusion

A lesion in the visual cortex or in a part of the visual pathway could prevent the fusion of the images of the two eyes.

Secondary Causes

Hereditary factors may affect each of the causes of strabismus. In addition, a precipitating condition, such as an injury, or an illness, may disrupt fusion, especially when it is weak or latent.

SENSORY CHANGES IN STRABISMUS

Before the age of six or seven, the sensory pattern of the eyes may be changed, and new adjustments are possible. Such changes and adjustments occur in strabismus. They include diplopia or double vision, suppression, and amblyopia exanopsia.

Diplopia or Double Vision

Diplopia means double vision, the seeing of the same object in two different locations at the same time. It results when the two eyes are not pointing at the same object. The image of the object seen by the straight eye falls on its fovea, but that seen by the deviating eye will fall on an extrafoveal retinal area and be related to some point away from the true position of the object seen by the straight eye. Thus, two images of the same object are observed. In addition, the fovea of the deviating eye will receive an image of some other object than that of primary observation, and the straight eye will observe this second object in an extrafoveal area. All objects are observed in two different positions and confusion results in the whole area of binocular vision due to superimposition.

Suppression

Since diplopia causes a confusion of images, the child will suppress or blot from consciousness the inferior visual image from the crossed eye. Suppression results in the development of a scotoma or blind spot in the macula of the crossed eye. Suppression is present only under binocular conditions.

Amblyopia Exanopsia

If monocular strabismus is not treated, suppression is likely to develop into loss of vision from disuse, amblyopia exanopsia, in the crossed eye. The visual acuity may be reduced to less than 20/200, an 80 percent or more visual loss.

In most cases amblyopia exanopsia is a preventable condition. Useful vision may be kept if the error in the crossed eye is corrected early enough in life, and the use of the crossed eye is encouraged by suitable exercises and by occulsion of the good eye, if necessary.

> The younger the child at the onset of strabismus, the easier and more rapid the onset of suppression. The earlier suppression starts, and the longer it is allowed to persist, the more profound and permanent the loss of vision. In infants, amblyopia can become deep within a week (Scheie and Albert, 1969, p. 157).

Other Sensory Changes

Eccentric Fixation

An amblyopic eye, when tested alone, may show an unsteady fixation when attempting to follow a light source. Furthermore, the eye will not point toward the light, but will appear to be looking in a different direction.

The unsteady fixation of the amblyopic eye may lead to a type of fixation with a part of the retina other than the fovea; this is known as eccentric fixation.

Anomalous Retinal Correspondence

An extrafoveal area of the crossed eye and the fovea of the straight eye may continue to send impulses to the brain. This is a primitive effort at binocular vision when strabismus is present, and is known as anomalous retinal correspondence. This condition is more likely to occur if the deviation is stable and of long standing. Also, it is more common among children who have a strong compulsion for fusion. Their fusional abilities can help overcome defects in each eye's picture. Anomalous retinal correspondence may become a serious barrier to a cure for strabismus.

EVALUATING THE STRABISMUS SUBJECT

The time for medical evaluation of strabismus is as soon as the condition is recognized. Complications of both a sensory and motor nature begin immediately for the subject. Various tests and examinations are given in evaluating the subject in order to know the treatment schedule to follow.

Muscle Balance

Tests are given to determine the muscular coordination for the straight-ahead direction and also for the detection of a rotation defect in other fields of gaze. Both monocular and binocular movements, as well as monocular and binocular fixations, are observed. The examiner looks for adaptive head positions, such as turning or tilting, that may be associated with strabismus.

Visual Acuity

The visual acuity of each eye separately and both together is evaluated. Refractive errors are measured. The eye specialist will use the ophthalmoscope to look into the interior of the eye for conditions, such as tumors or scars, that may be a contributing cause of strabismus.

History of the Condition

Since strabismus is commonly inherited as a dominant trait, the family history of the subject is important. Other factors should be known: age of onset, in infancy or childhood; whether the onset was gradual or sudden; and whether the deviation is always the same or varies.

Testing Devices

Two of the testing devices for strabismus will be considered, the cover-uncover test for muscle balance and the major amblyoscope for grades of fusion.

Cover-Uncover Test (Cover Test)

The cover-uncover test determines the presence of (1) a phoria which is a tendency of an eye to turn when fusion is interrupted, or (2) a tropia which is strabismus or squint. During the test, the subject looks at an object, such as a small light at eye level and 20 feet away for testing distance vision, and about 14 inches away for near vision.

In testing for phorias, one eye is occluded for several seconds to allow disruption of fusion. The occluder is removed so that both eyes are exposed. The observer watches the eye being uncovered for any motion.

Either eye may be tested first, but both should be observed because, although seldom encountered, it is possible to have a difference between the two sides, such as in double hyperphoria (tendency of both eyes to turn up) and in paresis (partial paralysis) of a muscle which is insufficient to show definite squint. Usually the phoria measured will be the same whether measured on right or left.

During the cover-uncover test for tropias, while the subject fixes on the test object, the cover is placed before one eye and the other is observed for motion. Each eye is checked separately. There is tropia if movement is observed on either or both sides. Movement on one side only is known as monocular strabismus; on both sides, alternating strabismus. In monocular (unilateral) strabismus, the fixing eye is easily determined.

Another use for the cover-uncover test is to measure the degree of deviation in both phorias and tropias. A prism, a glass or plastic wedge which changes the direction of light, is placed with its thicker edge or base in the direction opposite to the observed deviation. While shifting the cover from one eye to the other, the prism strength is varied until the one which neutralizes fixation motions of the eye is determined. This measures the amount of phoria or tropia.

The Major Amblyoscope

The major amblyoscope is a modified stereoscope which is used to evaluate the sensory status of the eye. The machine consists of two adjustable tubes which give a lighted image to each eye separately or together. The tubes can be moved up and down or sideways. The light source illuminates the images separately or together. A paired slide for each eye is placed at the end of each tube. The subject then looks into the amblyoscope.

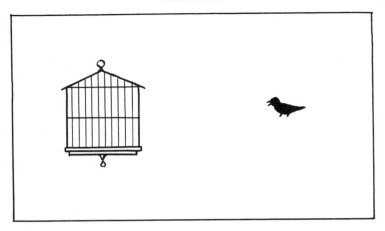

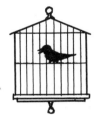

Figure 29. Grade 1 fusion or simultaneous binocular perception.

The amblyoscope measures three levels of binocular perception, usually referred to as grades of fusion.

Grade 1: Simultaneous binocular perception, the ability to see
with each eye at the same time.

This is binocular vision, but not fusion. Grade 1 requires that
the entire visual apparatus for each eye be functional up to the
higher perceptual centers.

Simultaneous binocular perception may be illustrated by pre-
senting two slides, each with a different picture, a bird and a
cage, for example (Figure 29). The correct response is to see the

cage and bird simultaneously, or the bird in the cage. If one object is not seen, the subject is suppressing in that eye.

Grade 2: Fusion of two images so that they are perceived as one.

This is the ability to merge two image perceptions, even though slightly dissimilar, into one image as interpreted by the higher centers. Fusion is developed to any great extent only in primates and possibly some birds. Grade 2 not only involves transmitting the image from the eye to the brain but also bringing the image to consciousness and coordinating the extraocular muscle movements.

Grade 2 fusion may be illustrated with two slides, each with a missing part; for example, each slide has two balls, each of which is incomplete (Figure 30). The correct response is three balls. If two or four balls are seen, the subject is not using both eyes together.

Grade 3: Depth perception or stereopsis.

Depth perception or stereopsis is a highly developed function of the brain that cannot operate unless Grades 1 and 2 are present. It is the ability to perceive depth through comparison of two slightly dissimilar images.

Grade 3 may be illustrated with two slides each with a chart with lines of similar characters, but with parallactic differences. When superimposed, one character in each line stands out. The correct response is calling the character that stands forward in each line. Failure is not being able to call the character that stands out; partial failure is being able to call correctly only some of the characters standing out.

The subject may need to take a minute or more to adjust his eyes so that he is able to perceive fusion and depth perception in the slides showing Grades 2 and 3 fusion. The three grades of fusion may be demonstrated by using a stereoscope with specially constructed cards.

In addition to being an instrument of evaluation, the major

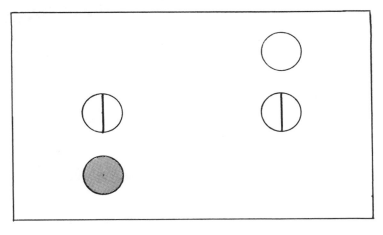

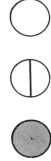

Figure 30. Grade 2 fusion.

amblyoscope is used in orthoptic therapy. The instrument may improve fixation, fusion, and rotational defects of the eyes.

PURPOSE OF STRABISMUS THERAPY AND METHODS USED

The defect in strabismus that usually demands attention is the deviating eye. The purpose of strabismus therapy is to obtain good vision in each eye, to have two straight eyes, and to gain binocular vision with fusion and stereopsis. Normal fusion is difficult to acquire unless the child had binocular vision before strabismus. Vaughan and Asbury (1977, p. 201) state that binocular vision is attained in fewer than half the cases of strabismus.

The methods used in therapy are (1) the occlusion of the straight eye to force the use of the crossed eye; (2) spectacles to correct refractive errors; (3) orthoptics to improve both monocular and binocular vision; and (4) surgery to straighten the crossed eye. It is important that the child receive treatment early, by six months of age, if the condition exists at that time.

Types of strabismus common to children, esotropia and exotropia, will be considered.

ESOTROPIA OR CONVERGENT STRABISMUS

Esotropia or convergent strabismus is the most common type. Comitant (concomitant) or nonparalytic esotropia is the usual kind found in infants and is characterized by showing the same angle of deviation in all directions of gaze. Noncomitant or paralytic strabismus is uncommon in children, but does occur.

Comitant or Nonparalytic Esotropia

Comitant esotropia is designated as nonaccommodative and accommodative.

NONACCOMMODATIVE ESOTROPIA. In nonaccommodative esotropia, the angle of deviation is not affected appreciably by accommodation. This type may be due to many different causes such as anomalous muscular anatomy, variations in innervation, and heredity. Two-thirds of the children with esotropia are nonaccommodative. Commonly the deviation appears at birth or by the first year.

Findings

Generally the mother is the first to notice the deviating eye, the only symptom. Either eye may deviate. There may be a refractive error. In monocular esotropia, the refractive error is usually more marked in the eye that deviates. In alternating esotropia, the refractive error is approximately the same in each eye. The vision becomes reduced in monocular deviations but not in alternating, since both eyes are being used.

Treatment

The straight eye is occluded, in order to prevent amblyopia in the crossed eye and to equalize visual acuity in the two eyes. Usually the earlier the deviation is found and occlusion started, the better will be the vision. The best results are obtained after the age of three. Weston (1980) notes that lenses to correct refractive errors, if needed, may be worn as early as one year of age, with the use of a head harness to keep the glasses in place.

The occlusive therapy may be combined with orthoptics in order to develop better binocular vision. When occlusion is discontinued, vision is likely to deteriorate unless the eye is straightened by glasses or surgery.

Pleoptics, a form of orthoptics, employs many techniques, often with dazzling lights, in order to disrupt eccentric fixation and bring about foveal fixation. However, pleoptics is considered by some ophthalmologists to be almost impractical because of expense, need for prolonged treatment, need for excellent attention and cooperation, and the danger of later relapse. This treatment is best for older children, from seven to fourteen years of age.

The object of surgery is to alter the position of the eye by moving the muscle insertions appropriately backward or forward. One method in nonaccommodative esotropia is to move the medial rectus muscle backward in order to weaken its pull, while the lateral rectus is moved forward to strengthen its pull.

Prognosis

Two or more operations may be necessary. Orthoptics just before, and again after surgery may help to improve vision, since the sensory adjustment is made more flexible because of the surgery.

ACCOMMODATIVE ESOTROPIA. In accommodative esotropia there are usually two diopters or more of hyperopia. About a third of childhood esotropia is of this type. Children with this condition must accommodate for distance vision; this is associated with convergence. At first the child may be able to compensate and control fusion, but when the hyperopia is severe in one eye, that eye is likely to turn inward. If the refractive error is the same in both eyes, the fixation may alternate between the eyes.

Findings

The symptom is a monocular or alternating deviation. The onset of accommodative esotropia is usually before the age of four. The accommodative faculty may not be well developed until that time.

Treatment

When treated early, purely accommodative esotropia may often be eliminated by wearing proper spectacles. The glasses relieve an excessive focusing effort in hyperopia. If the deviation is much greater for near than for distance, bifocals are recommended. The glasses are worn constantly, often for several years, or until the eyes remain straight without them. The strengthened fusion and decrease in hyperopia sometimes make this possible. In very young children, cycloplegic drugs may be used under careful supervision, instead of glasses, to paralyze accommodation during treatment.

If treatment is not begun until six months after the onset of accommodative esotropia, it may be necessary to use occlusion and have surgery.

Prognosis

When the treatment is started early, the prognosis is good. The subject may be expected to have good vision in each eye, straight eyes, and possibly good fusion.

Noncomitant or Paralytic Esotropia

Noncomitant or paralytic (paretic) strabismus in children is usually an esotropia caused by the paralysis of the lateral rectus muscle due to birth injury of the sixth nerve, the abducens. The nerve may partially recover from its damage.

EXOTROPIA OR DIVERGENT STRABISMUS

Exotropia in which an eye turns outward may be either monocular or alternating. The deviation is the same in all directions of gaze, and convergence is poor. Divergent strabismus is very seldom paralytic, and is less common in young children than convergent strabismus. Its incidence increases with age. Most cases start as a divergence excess. An exophoria may become an intermittent exotropia, and then a constant exotropia, if the subject receives no treatment.

Most young children with divergence excess do not have much of a refractive error. Myopia seems to increase the exotropia.

Intermittent Exotropia

More than half of the children with exotropia have the intermittent type. Often parents do not notice this condition since it occurs only when the child looks at something in the distance. The child may have fusion for near vision. Shutting one eye in bright light, such as sunlight, is a symptom frequently associated with intermittent exotropia.

The child usually does not develop amblyopia because he suppresses only part of the time. Vision may be normal. Glasses are prescribed if there is a refractive error. Surgery is usually required to correct intermittent exotropia.

Constant Exotropia

Constant exotropia is rarely a congenital defect, although it may be present at birth. It may occur when intermittent exotropia progresses to constant, or this condition may take place following the loss of vision in one eye.

Glasses are required if there is a refractive error. Occlusion, orthoptics, or pleoptics may be used, but surgery is usually necessary. In this operation the lateral rectus muscle is weakened while the medial rectus is strengthened.

Educational Implications

Occasionally a child with strabismus, who must wear an occluder, attends a resource room for the partially seeing for a short time. This makes it more comfortable for him as he uses his amblyopic eye. In such a room he receives attention to his particular need. The teacher uses special methods and materials with him. These may include better lighting, large type books if needed, an opportunity for eye rest, and less tension in the room than in a regular classroom.

Strabismus is not as common as formerly in the Detroit area, and probably throughout the country. Children are being treated at an earlier age before the strabismus becomes firmly established. This early treatment has been brought about by such factors as preschool vision testing, advice from doctors and health agencies, and literature stressing the importance of immediate referral.

Strabismus usually does not cause headaches or eyestrain. However, the emotional aspects may be devastating. A child is almost always sensitive about his crossed eye. He may be withdrawn or display antisocial behavior. For this reason it is important to have the eye cosmetically corrected before he enters school.

The teacher of the visually impaired has specialized knowledge of strabismus and its effects on the child. He or she should explain to parents the need for referral to an ophthalmologist for early treatment. Also, the teacher should give this information to other faculty members as needed.

REFERENCES

Allen, James H. *May's Diseases of the Eye.* 23rd ed. Baltimore: Williams & Wilkins, 1963.

Jampolsky, Arthur. "Strabismus." In L. Byerly Holt (Ed.), *Pediatric Ophthalmology.* Philadelphia: Lea and Febiger, 1964, 210-259.

Liebman, Sumner D. and Gellis, Sydney S. (Eds.). *The Pediatrician's Ophthalmology.* St. Louis: C. V. Mosby, 1966.

Scheie, Harold G. and Albert, Daniel M. *Adler's Textbook of Ophthalmology.* 8th ed. Philadelphia: W. B. Saunders, 1969.

Vaughan, Daniel and Asbury, Taylor. *General Ophthalmology.* 8th ed. Los Altos: Lange Medical Publications, 1977.

Chapter 9

CAUSES OF VISUAL IMPAIRMENT IN THE SCHOOLS; INTERPRETING EYE EXAMINATION REPORTS

DATA FROM A LARGE city school system should enable the prospective teacher of the visually impaired to know what eye pathologies to expect in his or her program. For this reason, the following information is presented.

Preschool children or children in the Detroit Schools are considered for the special education program after they have obtained a written medical report from their professional eye specialist or an eye clinic. Prospective candidates and their parents are then given an appointment at the School Vision Clinic.

The Clinic is operated by the Detroit Public Schools. A specially assigned ophthalmologist and the supervisor of the program for the visually impaired are present at all clinic sessions to certify and admit eligible children. The ophthalmologist gives the child a vision test, reviews the eye specialist's examination report, and indicates the primary eye condition. The supervisor has pertinent reports either from the preschool teacher-consultant or from the school the child attends. On the basis of medical and school information, a decision is made regarding placement.

Entrants to the program are classified as either partially seeing or blind. Generally speaking, the partially seeing are defined as being able to use their vision as the main avenue of learning. They have approximately 64 percent of normal vision or less; their corrected visual acuity is 20/70 or below. The blind are those unable to read print either because their corrected vision is inadequate, or they have no vision at all.

CAUSES OF VISUAL IMPAIRMENTS

Many low-visioned and blind children have more than one diagnosis of eye difficulties. Only the primary eye problem as indicated by the ophthalmologist at the Vision Clinic is indicated here.

Partially Seeing Children

Table I shows the primary eye conditions of 240 partially seeing children in Special Education at present. Of these students, fifty-four are in the teacher counselor program and the remainder in resource rooms.

The figures in Table I indicate that the chief cause of low vision is myopia. Nystagmus ranks second and cataract, mostly congenital, ranks third.

Table II gives the primary eye conditions of 927 partially seeing children during the period of 1948-63.

A comparison of Tables I and II clearly indicates that the limited vision in both periods is traceable to the same chief causes, namely myopia, nystagmus and cataract. The proportion of children with myopia has increased considerably, from 40.0 percent in the 1948-63 period to 48.3 percent at the present time. Further comparison of the two tables shows that at present albinism accounts for 8.8 percent of the low vision; in the earlier

TABLE I

PRIMARY EYE CONDITIONS OF 240 PARTIALLY SEEING CHILDREN IN
PRESENT ENROLLMENT, 1980

Eye Condition	*No. of Children*	*Percent of Children*
Myopia	116	48.3
Nystagmus	35	14.6
Cataract	23	9.5
Albinism	21	8.8
Hyperopia	9	3.8
Retinal degeneration	8	3.3
Retinitis pigmentosa	6	2.5
Dislocated lens	4	1.7
Optic atrophy	4	1.7
Infrequent causes*	14	5.8
Total†	240	100.0

* The infrequent causes occurred in less than 1 percent of the cases. They consisted of the following defects and diseases: choroidal scars, corneal scars, glaucoma, keratoconus, megalocornea, and ptosis.

† Information from Tables I and III was supplied by Miss Shirley Gustafson, Supervisor, Program for the Visually Impaired, Detroit Public Schools.

TABLE II

PRIMARY EYE CONDITIONS OF 927 PARTIALLY SEEING CHILDREN,
1948-63

Eye Condition	No. of Children	Percent of Children
Myopia	371	40.0
Cataract	115	12.4
Nystagmus	89	9.7
Hyperopia	83	9.0
Strabismus	55	5.9
Albinism	35	3.6
Retrolental fibroplasia	32	3.5
Infrequent causes*	147	15.9
Total†	927	100.0

* Occur in less than 3.5 percent of cases.
† Information in Tables II and IV is from Kirk (1965).

study, 3.6 percent. Albinism affects dark-skinned races more than light-skinned. During recent years many families of dark-skinned races, particularly from the Near East, have settled in Detroit. This fact appears to account for the increase of albinism in the schools.

Blind Children

The eye conditions resulting in blindness are somewhat different from those causing low vision. Table III shows the primary

TABLE III

PRIMARY EYE CONDITIONS OF 46 BLIND CHILDREN IN PRESENT
ENROLLMENT, 1980

Eye Condition	No. of Children	Percent of Children
Congenital Cataract	10	21.8
Optic Atrophy	7	15.2
Nystagmus	6	13.0
Retrolental Fibroplasia	5	10.9
Retinoblastoma	4	8.7
Congenital Glaucoma	3	6.5
Retinitis Pigmentosa	3	6.5
Cortical Blindness	2	4.4
Infrequent causes*	6	13.0
Total	46	100.0

* The infrequent causes occurred in less than 2.5 percent of the cases. They consisted of the following defects and diseases: atrophic hypoplastic disc, microphthalmos, myopia, neurofibromatosis, and retinal scars.

causes of blindness of the forty-six children in the present enrollment.

These data indicate that cataract is the chief cause of blindness. Optic atrophy is the second major cause, and nystagmus, mostly congenital, is the third.

Table IV showing the primary causes of blindness during the 1948-63 period, is included for comparison.

As indicated in Table IV, the primary cause of blindness during 1948-63 was retrolental fibroplasia. The second and third were congenital cataract and congenital glaucoma. During that period, retrolental fibroplasia accounted for more than half of the children in the program. There has been a dramatic decrease in this disease to the present 10.9 percent. There has likewise been a decrease in microphthalmos. Possibly some of the microphthalmos was due to retrolental fibroplasia.

The proportion of children in the present enrollment with optic atrophy and congenital cataracts has increased since the earlier 1948-63 period. In addition, there is now a higher percentage of children with retinoblastoma. More persons with this highly hereditary malignancy are now surviving to adulthood, marriage, and children.

Hatfield (1975) has completed another study of the causes of blindness in school children. Comparisons between her study and the foregoing material cannot be made. Her study includes only children with 0 vison to 80 percent visual loss. This material

TABLE IV
PRIMARY EYE CONDITIONS OF 170 BLIND CHILDREN, 1948-63

Eye Condition	No. of Children	Percent of Children
Retrolental Fibroplasia	88	51.8
Congenital Cataract	13	7.7
Optic Atrophy	11	6.3
Congenital Glaucoma	13	7.7
Cortical Blindness	7	4.2
Microphthalmos	11	6.3
Infrequent causes*	27	16.0
Total	170	100.0

* Occur in less than 4.2 percent.

includes children from 0 vision to 36 percent visual loss, and separates them into blind and partially seeing.

Hatfield's study contains much valuable information for teachers and for parents with visually impaired children. Hatfield (1975, p. 11) states that prenatal influence was responsible for the greatest amount of blindness, one-half of all blind students. Of these, 83 percent were hereditary or genetic in origin. The remaining 17 percent in the prenatal category were congenital, but without a definitely known cause. It is thought that such factors as infectious diseases or the use of drugs or medications during pregnancy may be responsible.

Hatfield's study reported an increase in the prevalence of neoplasms but a decrease in blindness from infectious diseases and injuries.

INTERPRETING EYE EXAMINATION REPORT FORMS

After a child has been approved for admittance and enters a program for the visually impaired, the special teacher receives a copy of his eye examination report. In Detroit, there is one report from the child's eye specialist and another from the ophthalmologist at the School Vision Clinic. Usually the information supplied, along with the teacher's own background in eye pathology, is sufficient to know how to adjust the child's program to his visual needs. Occasionally when further information is necessary, the special teacher will contact the department supervisor, or the child's eye specialist, depending upon school policy.

Different school systems have devised examination report forms which are completed by the child's eye specialist. The form developed by the National Society for the Prevention of Blindness, "Eye Report for Children with Visual Problems," is periodically evaluated and changed, and is widely used; it is reproduced here (p. 199). When this form is completely filled out by the child's eye specialist, the information is invaluable to the teacher. In addition, the completed form is helpful and even indispensable in research aimed at reducing and preventing low vision and blindness everywhere. Comments will be made about each of the parts of the National Society's form.

The top part of the form is necessary to furnish background information for the special teacher and for future studies. The report is confidential.

A. *Name in Full:*

Both the middle and last names are necessary. They may reveal a blood relationship to other persons with similar vision problems.

B. *Sex:*

The first name does not always indicate the sex of the child. Some eye conditions are more common among males; others, among females. A number of diseases and defects are sex-linked or have a tendency to be more common among either males or females. Color blindness is sex-linked, and is more common in males. Retrolental fibroplasia is not sex-linked; however, it is more prevalent in females. This disease is thought to be associated with the lower birth weight of the female.

C. *Race:*

Some eye diseases are reported to be more common among certain races and ethnic groups. For example, degenerative myopia is reported to be more common among the Chinese, Arabs, and Jewish persons. This fact can only be confirmed by collecting more data.

D. *Complete Address Including County and State:*

This information is needed for obvious reasons.

E. *Date of Birth and Grade:*

The date of birth and grade level are indicators of whether or not the child is progressing at the normal or expected rate in school.

F. *School and Address:*

The school keeps records for a long period of time as permanent records. This is especially helpful for the child who moves often.

I. History

A. *Probable age of onset of vision impairment, right eye and left eye:*

An early age of onset is frequently considered more hazardous for good vision than if the defect or disease occurred at a later age. For example, the earlier infantile glaucoma becomes manifest, the less favorable is the prognosis. An early onset of strabismus may prevent the development of binocular vision and fusion.

The age of onset in both the right and left eyes is requested because some conditions may affect only one eye while others affect both eyes, but at different times. Retinoblastoma is a disease that may affect one eye or both eyes.

Low vision or blindness imposes a handicap on the sensory data available to the child. When a child is thus afflicted at a very early age, he is almost certain to be retarded in his development of concepts. The early years of a child's life are the period when intelligence develops most rapidly.

B. *Severe ocular infections, injuries, operations, if any; with age at time of occurrence:*

Certain infections, injuries, or operations may cause further vision problems years later. Preschool operations for congenital cataract occasionally result in retinal detachment after the young person has reached junior or senior high school.

C. *Has the pupil's ocular condition occurred in any blood relative(s)? If so, what relationship?*

Many eye conditions of visually impaired children are inherited. Generally the closer the relationship of a person with a hereditary eye defect or disease, the more likely the child is to have it. Infants born to parents with a family history of genetic visual defects should be carefully examined periodically by an ophthalmologist. In certain instances, it is possible to interrupt or change the course of the disease before it has affected vision.

II. Measurements

A. *Visual acuity, both distant and near, without correction, with best correction, and with low vision aid in the right eye, left eye, and both eyes. The prescription for glasses and the date of examination are requested.*

The vision indicated by the examiner is what the teacher may expect the child to have when he enters the class or special program. However, young children as well as those who have not worn prescribed glasses, may have an improvement in vision after wearing their glasses for a while. This is due to a number of factors, such as the stimulation of the visual centers of the brain by receiving a sharper image, increased motivation, and better concentration.

When a child seems to have better vision than indicated on the report, the teacher may check the visual acuity. This is done by using the Snellen Test Chart to measure the distant vision and a near-point chart, such as the Jaeger, for near visual acuity.

Occasionally there is very little difference in visual acuity with or without glasses. For example, a child with nystagmus may have only a small refractive error. However, in addition to correcting that error, the glasses may have a steadying effect on the nystagmus.

The prescription gives the special teacher additional information. It indicates if the refractive error is severe. The date of the prescription should be less than a year old if a child is being considered for special education.

It should be noted that not all children, no matter how visually impaired, profit from wearing glasses.

B. *If glasses are to be worn, were safety lenses prescribed in plastic or in tempered glass?*

Law now requires that all glasses have safety lenses. If the lenses are of plastic, they will scratch more easily than do those of tempered glass. Children's glasses should have strong frames.

It may be necessary for the special teacher to discuss the care of glasses with both the children and their parents. This includes keeping the glasses clean and straight, using both hands to remove or replace the glasses, and storing them so that the lenses will not be scratched.

C. *If low vision aid is prescribed, specify type and recommendation for use:*

This is valuable information for the teacher as he or she encourages and helps the child to become proficient in the use of the low vision aid. Usually such aids are not prescribed for an early elementary child. The aid is difficult for the young child to handle and he is frustrated by the narrow field of vision. However, there are exceptions to this generalization.

D. *Field of Vision: Is there a limitation? If so, record results of test on chart on back of form. What is the widest diameter (in degrees) of remaining visual field in the right eye, and in the left eye?*

When the peripheral field is greatly limited or restricted, the teacher will expect the child to have difficulty in walking and moving about since it is the peripheral vision that keeps one oriented to his environment. The special teacher will know that certain eye diseases, such as some glaucomas and retinitis pigmentosa, are likely to result in a restricted peripheral field.

If central vision is largely destroyed, and the child has mainly peripheral vision, he will have extremely low acuity. The child will have great difficulty in reading or doing close eye work. In addition, it may appear that such a child is not looking at the person to whom he is speaking. This is due to the fact that he does not have central fixation.

E. *Is there impaired color perception? If so, for what colors?*

Knowledge of this disability will be helpful to the teacher as the young child is taught the different colors. Incomplete color blindness is known as dyschromatopsia. This is the common type of color blindness that affects about 8 percent of males and 0.45 percent of females. Usually the person confuses reds, greens, and blues, but has normal visual acuity. Dyschromatopsia is inherited as a sex-linked recessive trait.

The complete loss of color vision is known as achromatopsia. Colors of the spectrum are seen in tones of white-gray-black, usually gray. The tones appear as different degrees of brightness. Achromatopsia is a very rare condition that is associated with low visual acuity.

Detroit special teachers have noticed that children who have such low vision that they are borderline between blind and partially seeing have great difficulty in distinguishing colors even when those colors are clear and strong. Such children have degenerative diseases of the retina or optic nerve.

III. Cause of Blindness or Vision Impairment

A. *Present ocular condition(s) responsible for vision impairment:*

Many visually impaired children have more than one eye disease or defect, but there is a primary one, as indicated in Tables I through IV of this chapter. Knowing the primary cause gives the teacher more understanding of the child's background and what can be expected of him. For example, a child with aphakia may not have had the necessary operation until he became of school age. Consequently, before the operation, he was deprived of many learning experiences which vision normally supplies.

B. *Preceding ocular condition, if any, which led to present condition:*

An example of such a condition is degenerative myopia which caused the retina to become detached, or retrolental fibroplasia which caused microphthalmos.

C. *Etiology (underlying cause) of ocular condition primarily responsible for vision impairment:*

Often these are prenatal conditions with the great majority being genetic in origin.

D. *If etiology is injury or poisoning, indicate circumstances and kind of object or poison involved:*

This information will increase the teacher's understanding of the child and the injury and pain that he has had. In addition, such data are needed for research in the prevention of blindness.

IV. Prognosis and Recommendations

A. *Is pupil's vision impairment considered to be stable, deteriorating, capable of improvement, uncertain:*

This information is useful to the special teacher as he or she works with the individual child and assists in the planning of his further schooling. The teacher's background in eye pathology will be helpful in knowing the prognosis of the disease or defect.

B. *What treatment is recommended, if any?*

Treatment may include glasses, exercises, surgery, and/or

medication. When the child requires glasses, the teacher may need to follow through to be certain they are obtained and then worn. As a general rule, teachers do not put medication in children's eyes. If the child is too young to take care of this, the teacher will contact the school nurse or school principal regarding the medication, depending upon school policy.

C. *When is re-examination recommended?*

Annual eye examinations are usually recommended, but this may vary. In Detroit almost all children in programs for the visually impaired have an annual eye examination unless they are permanently blind.

D. *Glasses not needed, to be worn constantly, for close work only, other:*

Usually visually impaired children who have glasses need to wear them all the time. Children, especially when they are young, who frequently take their glasses off and put them on, either bend the frames or lose the glasses.

E. *Lighting requirements: Average, better than average, less than average:*

Many visually impaired children can function under average illumination. However, better than average lighting increases the sharpness of images for most of the children. A few such as those with albinism, aniridia, and central cataract may have better visual acuity under less than average lighting.

F. *Use of eyes: unlimited or limited, as follows:*

Most ophthalmologists do not put limits on the use of children's and young person's eyes since vision develops with use. However, after an injury or recent operation, there may be some restrictions.

G. *Physical activity: restricted or unrestricted, as follows:*

Some eye conditions, such as degenerative myopia or displaced lenses, may require restricted physical activity. In other instances, such as advanced retinitis pigmentosa, the disease itself may restrict the young person's physical activity. When the ophthalmologist makes the decision about restricting physical activity, it removes that responsibility from the teacher and school. The school is careful to follow the doctor's directions.

The bottom part of the National Society's eye form requests the address to which the completed form is to be sent, date of the eye examination, signature of the examiner, his degree, and address. When the person is examined at a clinic the name of the clinic as well as the clinic number given to the child is needed.

When the examiner is a physician, the degree following his name will be M.D. for medical doctor. This usually means that the examiner is an ophthalmologist, a physician who is a specialist in diseases of the eye. When the examiner is an optometrist, the degree following his name will be O.D. for doctor of optometry. The optometrist is a licensed person who mainly measures refractive errors and muscle disturbances and prescribes glasses. To avoid confusion, the optician should be mentioned here. An optician is a technician who grinds lenses for eye glasses, fits them into frames, and adjusts the frames to the wearer.

The back of the National Society's form (p. 200) contains three headings: Preferred Visual Acuity Notations, Table of Approximate Equivalent Visual Acuity Notations, and Field of Vision.

Preferred Visual Acuity Ratings

The Snellen Test Chart with which everyone is familiar, uses standardized letters (or the symbol E) of various sizes which are displayed at a standard distance with lighting of uniform brightness. Usually the subject reads a Snellen chart at a distance of 20 feet (6 meters). At this distance rays of light from an object are practically parallel, and accommodation is not necessary.

Visual acuity is recorded in the form of a fraction. The numerator (top number) is the distance of the subject to the chart; the denominator (bottom number) is the size of the test number. Vision of 20/20 means that the subject is seeing at a distance of 20 feet what the normal eye sees at 20 feet. A vision of 20/100 means that the subject is seeing at 20 feet what the normal eye can see at a distance of 100 feet.

If the subject must move to 10 feet from the test chart in order to see the largest letter, his vision is recorded as 10/200.

Table of Approximate Equivalent Visual Acuity Notations

This section is self-explanatory.

Field of Vision

The normal field of vision for the left eye and for the right eye is indicated. If there is a limitation in either or both fields, the examiner records it here.

SUMMARY OF RELATIONSHIP BETWEEN VISUAL ACUITY AND VISUAL EFFICIENCY

Distance (Snellen Chart)

Distance Visual Acuity	% Visual Efficiency
20/20	100
20/25	95
20/30	91.5
20/40	85
20/50	75
20/70	64
20/80	60
20/100	50
20/160	30
20/200	20
20/400 or 10/200	10

Near (Jaeger Test Type)

Near Visual Acuity	% Visual Efficiency
1	100
2	100
3	90
6	50
7	40
11	15
14	5

Low Vision Measurements*

CF Counts fingers, usually at 3 feet
HM Hand Movements
PLL Perceives and localizes light
LP Perceives, but does not localize light
No LP No light perception.

* "Low vision measurements are, at most, only approximate. I have always considered 3/200 to be about the same as counting fingers at 3 feet. Even then one is hardly measuring macular vision at that distance; the angle involved in seeing the 20/200 E at 3 feet involves some extrafoveal vision" (Weston, 1980, p. 19).

REFERENCES

Chalkley, Thomas. *Your Eyes.* Springfield: Charles C Thomas, Publisher, 1974.

Hatfield, Elizabeth M. "Why Are They Blind?" *Sightsaving Review,* 1975, 45, 3-22.

Kirk, Edith C. "Changes and Trends in the Characteristics of Children in Classes for the Visually Handicapped." Unpublished Doctoral Dissertation, Wayne State University, 1965.

Vail, Derrick. *The Truth About Your Eyes.* New York: Farrar, Straus and Cudahy, 1959.

Chapter 10

VISION SCREENING DURING SCHOOL AND PRESCHOOL YEARS

TODAY A VAST AMOUNT of information is known about the eyes and vision, and many eye specialists and clinics are available to care for and correct vision problems. It follows that all children should have an eye examination and necessary treatment during preschool years so that they may enter school with the best possible vision. The school should keep a record of the vision examination.

All children and young persons, as they progress through school, should have eye examinations at regular intervals. Eye problems, many of which are correctable with spectacles, increase with age.

> We find that the prevalence of visual defects among children increases year by year throughout their school life. Defects of vision among children in high school reach 35%. (Radke and Blackhurst, 1978, pp. 104-5).

Many states require that some type of vision screening be given in their schools. The State of Michigan has done much more than this. In 1968 two groups of eye specialists, ophthalmologists and optometrists, united to support the passage of a legislative bill, Public Act 282, which makes preschool vision testing mandatory. This bill requires that every child pass a screening test or have an examination by an eye specialist before first entering school. Public Act 282 was supported and augmented by Part 93 of the Public Health Code of 1978 which requires that parents registering a child for the first time in kindergarten or first grade present a certificate of vision testing or screening. This legislation has greatly increased the amount of vision screening throughout the state.

Screening the vision of preschool children is very important. Early detection and treatment of eye problems may not only save the child's vision but also enable him to make a better adjustment on entering school. The National Society for the Prevention of Blindness recommends three screenings of the preschool child.

> As a minimum, eye screening should be done at three age levels: the newborn, six months, and three to five years (Hatfield, 1979, p. 83).

Since 1957 Michigan has been successfully screening the vision of preschool and kindergarten children in the three-to-five age-group. The program received its impetus from the fact that certain children were entering school with little or no sight in one eye. A crossed or deviating eye, or a refractive error in one eye, can cause suppression followed by loss of vision through disuse.

The results of preschool screening in Michigan, as well as in other parts of the country, are evident. It is now less common to see school-age children with uncorrected strabismus; many have been treated before entering school.

THE PURPOSE OF SCREENING TESTS

Screening tests determine the extent to which a subject's visual performance compares to a standard. They provide a step toward securing professional eye examinations for children who need them. The tests do not prove that a subject either has or does not have a defect; the eye specialist makes this decision. Furthermore, a child may pass a screening test and still have a vision defect that cannot be observed; for example, early findings of retinitis pigmentosa.

Many tests have been developed for screening vision, and different persons, including school nurses, teachers, and parents, have administered the tests. The Michigan program has had outstanding success and will be discussed here.

ESTABLISHING STANDARDS AND PROCEDURES

The Vision Section of the Michigan Department of Public Health is responsible for establishing standards and procedures for the screening of both school and preschool vision throughout the state. Before setting up the program, vision consultants from the Department of Health conferred with eye specialists.

The consultants and specialists determined the equipment and tests to be used, the procedures for screening, the referral standards to be followed, and the forms to develop for contacting parents and eye specialists. At periodic intervals the vision consultants and eye specialists meet to review procedures and standards, and to make modifications in the program.

Local public health departments conduct the program in their areas; contacting the schools or homes of children; employing certified vision technicians to do the actual screening; and doing follow-up work on those children, both school-age and preschool, who do not pass the screening tests.

CONTACTING SCHOOLS AND HOMES

The local department of health has the responsibility of informing parents about the vision screening program. For school-age pupils, the health department contacts the school where the screening will take place. Preschool children are not as easily located.

The health department obtains information concerning preschool children from the census records of the intermediate school office; also, from public schools and nursery schools in the area. Letters are then sent to all parents of the children informing them about the screening program.

Parents are requested to call the department of health if they wish to have their children included in the program. Parents who call for an appointment are sent a form entitled "Preschool Vision Screening Record," a copy of which is reproduced here (p. 198), and a training card for practicing the visual acuity test with their child. Parents are requested to complete the top part of the form concerning name and address and also a section entitled a Brief Eye History. The parents return the form when their child is screened.

USING VISION TECHNICIANS

Persons who do the screening are known as vision technicians. Frequently they are nurses who have a special concern for eye problems. The technicians are carefully trained and certified for their work by the Vision Section of the Michigan Department of

Public Health. Periodically they are invited to participate in workshops or conferences in order to upgrade their knowledge and skills.

There are many advantages in using certified technicians. They are thoroughly familiar with the instrument used for screening, how to operate it, and how to interpret the results. All technicians use the same procedures in screening and in reporting. This uniformity makes it possible to measure the results of their work. If technicians cannot be used in screening school-age pupils, the Vision Section of the Department of Public Health recommends that screening be limited to the Snellen Chart.

Most technicians screen from sixty-five to seventy-five children or young persons a day when administering the Michigan Vision Test, as described on page 155.

In testing preschool children, the technician must be friendly, calm, and positive in order to establish rapport and communication, and thereby obtain accurate results from the screening. The technician must be patient throughout the testing period. Such characteristics help to do away with a young child's short attention span, apprehension, and fatigue.

During the average day the technician screens about thirty-five children, approximately half as many as school-age pupils.

BASIC SCREENING TESTS

The screening tests for school-age pupils and preschool children have essentially the same purpose, but use different procedures.

School-age Pupils

The three basic screening tests are (1) an obvious sign of an eye problem, (2) a visual acuity test such as the Snellen Chart, and (3) a battery of tests known as the Michigan Vision Test. Ideally all three methods should be used. If a pupil does not pass any one of these tests, referral is made through parents to an eye specialist.

SIGNS OF EYE PROBLEMS. Parents, technicians, nurses, and teachers are likely to notice conditions which indicate the need for professional eye examinations: a crossed eye, nystagmus, ptosis, and unequal pupils (anisocoria). Other signs which are sometimes significant may include tenseness of the body when trying to see, unusual irritability, frowning, tearing, and itching or hurting eyes. Children with serious reading problems are included in this category.

The teacher observes the behavior and complaints of children in a variety of learning situations and can sometimes identify those with visual defects. One such child may hold the book close to his eyes and tilt the head while reading; another may squint or shut one eye when looking at distant objects; and still another may walk over-cautiously or stumble easily. Certain children with eye problems may complain of dizziness, headache, blurring, or pain in the eyes. If such behavior or complaints persist, the children should have professional eye examinations even though screening test results are within normal range.

VISUAL ACUITY. The Snellen Chart, when used exactly as directed, is an accurate means of screening for visual acuity. Teachers, nurses, or vision technicians do this screening. When a pupil does not pass, retesting is done a week later before parents are advised of the need for an eye examination.

MICHIGAN VISION TEST. The Michigan Vision Test is designed for persons six years of age and older. In administering the test, a stereoscopic instrument is used. The instrument is compact and may be placed on a table during the screening. When necessary it can be used in a small room. Self-contained lighting in the instrument assures standardized illumination. The testing charts are photographically reduced in size and placed on slides; thereby a twenty-foot distance is effectively simulated. The pictures seen by each eye are isolated.

The local department of public health sets up schedules for the vision technicians and informs schools regarding the time of screening. Before the actual screening, the technician gives an explanation of the tests to a group of children. Naturally children in early elementary grades will require more explanations and demonstrations. The technician may need to practice with some children before the screening.

The four tests in the Michigan Battery are given in the following order: near phoria, far phoria, visual acuity, and plus lens.

Near Phoria

The near phoria test is administered only to pupils in grades 9 through 12. It is a test for muscle balance at near point, approximately 14 inches. On the slide a white outline of a rectangular box is presented to one eye; a red ball is presented to the other. The vertical dimensions of the box are determined by the prescribed limits of the vertical phoria (hyperphoria or hypophoria) and the horizontal dimensions by the limits of the lateral phoria (esophoria or exophoria). If the pupil sees the ball in the box, he is using both eyes within normal limits, and passes. If he sees the ball outside the box, he may not be using both eyes together; he does not pass and is given a retest a week later. Such retests reduce unnecessary referrals.

The relationship seen between the box and the ball determines the amount of muscle imbalance. Pupils fail if they need corrections for the following amounts of prism diopters: 6 of esophoria, 8 of exophoria, and 1½ of hyperphoria.

Far Phoria

The far phoria test for muscle balance, at a simulated 20-foot distance, is administered to all pupils. The same type of slides are used as in the near phoria. Again, if the ball is outside the box, the pupil does not pass and is retested a week later. Pupils fail if they need corrections for the following amounts of prism diopters: 6 of esophoria, 4 of exophoria, and 1½ of hyperphoria.

Visual Acuity

The Snellen E test for visual acuity is incorporated into the instrument used. The test identifies a large number of children and young persons who have defects, and its findings have a high correlation with the findings of eye specialists for distance visual acuity. Each eye is tested separately. If the pupil misses the 20/30 line with either eye, he does not pass. A retest is given a week later before referral is made through parents to an eye specialist.

The Snellen E test may not find the hyperopic subject because children have a high reserve of accommodative power, and some may have been using it as they read the Snellen E test.

Plus Lens

The plus lens test is designed to identify children with an excessive amount of hyperopia. During this test the pupil is asked to read the 20/20 line of Snellen E symbols while looking through a pair of plus 1.75 D spherical lenses. For pupils with normal vision, the E symbols become blurred, and their visual acuity score is reduced. For pupils with hyperopia, the lens replaces accommodation, and their visual acuity score may improve. If a pupil is able to read four to six of the symbols with either eye while looking through the plus lens, he does not pass and is retested a week later. An exception to this are pupils in grades 7 to 12. It is the opinion of eye specialists that these older pupils who do not pass the first time should be referred for professional eye care.

A failure may indicate that the child or young person has hyperopia or a problem of accommodation that may make reading and close eye work difficult and fatiguing. Those who do not pass the plus lens test may have other educational problems. They comprise only 1 or 2 percent of the school population.

Color Vision, on Request

Color vision tests are sometimes added to the vision screening program. In Michigan these tests are now administered to pupils at the kindergarten and junior high school levels, if requested by a school. During kindergarten most of the child's program is color oriented. In junior high school, color discrimination may be important as a young person determines his future vocation.

Such tests are usually administered at the same time as the vision screening. Both functional and diagnostic tests are used. All are designed to detect deficiencies in the primary colors and shades thereof. In order to insure accuracy, the tests must be given in daylight or in illumination by special bulbs that produce light of all spectral lengths.

The functional test consists of a number of easily manipulated cards which are similar in size, shape, reflectance, and saturation. Only the colors vary. During the functional test, the subject is asked to name colors, match colors, pick out colors, and recognize colors that are alike and different. This test is most appropriate for kindergarten and early elementary children but may be used in junior high grades.

The diagnostic test consists of pseudo-isochromatic test plates usually bound together in book form. The plates have symbols made up of dots of the various colors printed on a background of dots in a confusion of colors. The symbols are not discernible by subjects with color perception defects. The diagnostic test can be used to indicate the type of defective color vision and the intensity of the defect.

Children show a wide range of ability in their discrimination of color. When the testing is completed, the teacher is informed of the child's capability in color discrimination.

At the present time eye specialists and educators generally recommend that a color vision test be given at least twice, once in kindergarten or first grade, and again in later elementary.

Preschool Children

The five basic screening tests for preschool children are administered in the following order: (1) visual acuity, (2) corneal reflection, (3) cover-uncover, (4) an eye problem as indicated in the Brief History section of the "Preschool Vision Screening Record," and (5) signs of eye problems. Children who do not pass the visual acuity test are retested a week later, when possible.

VISUAL ACUITY. An instrument designed especially for preschool and kindergarten children is used for screening visual acuity. The device is compact, self-illuminating, and is adaptable to a relatively small space. It is set on a table or chair in order to be at eye level of the child being screened. The instrument uses a modified Snellen E at 10 feet; a 10-foot distance provides for good communication with the child. The E points to different objects or symbols with which young children are familiar: car, hat, sock, and ball. All the symbols have a similar overall configuration.

The training card sent the parents is a small reproduction of the visual acuity test. Instructions on the back of the card show the parents how to practice with their child. This practice gives the children confidence and even enthusiasm when they take the test.

The technician also does some practicing with the children using both a training card and an occluder in preparation for testing the eyes separately as well as together. First both eyes are tested together, then each eye separately. The three-and-four-year-olds do not pass if they miss the 20/40 symbol; the five-year olds, if they miss the 20/30 symbol.

Vision test cards are used with children too young or too immature for the instrument. In one set there are twelve cards to test the level of visual acuity. This set has the same symbols as those on the instrument. The screening may be done by using four symbols, three symbols, or even two. The child may name the object, point to it, match it, or otherwise indicate a choice. The same pass or fail levels are used as in the vision screening instrument.

The visual acuity test is considered the best one for mass screening. It identifies many children in need of eye care, and readily detects most significant refractive errors. However, the visual acuity test may miss one-eyed vision loss due to a muscle problem, because in the preschool test, only one symbol of the E chart is exposed at a time. An isolated symbol is easier to discriminate than a line of symbols as used in the school vision testing.

CORNEAL REFLECTION TEST. The corneal reflection test is for muscle balance; the test also enables the technician to observe conditions, such as nystagmus and blepharitis. During the corneal reflection test, the technician holds a penlight about 13 inches from the child's eye while he (the child) looks at the light. In normal eyes the reflection of light will be in the center of both pupils. The child does not pass if the reflection is in the center of one pupil, but off-center in the other.

COVER-UNCOVER TEST. The routine of the cover-uncover test, as devised by Radke and Blackhurst (1978, pp. 101-2), is another test for muscle balance. It allows fusion to be disrupted and careful observation by the vision technician can detect a phoria. The test consists of six steps in which an occluder is used: the occluder is placed in front of the child's right eye, then moved to the left eye, and then to the left of both eyes; next the occluder is again placed in front of the left eye, then moved to the right eye, and finally to the right of both eyes.

A near-point cover-uncover test is given while the child looks at something small (a coin, for example) held in the technician's hand 14 to 16 inches away. A far-point test is given while the child looks at something (a toy, for example) 20 or more feet away.

In both near and distance testing, if there is any movement or shift of the eye being uncovered, the child does not pass the test.

BRIEF EYE HISTORY. The Brief Eye History section in the "Preschool Vision Screening Record" has two questions. The first asks if the child has ever been examined by an eye specialist. The second asks if, when the child is ill or tired, do his eyes appear crossed, or does one eye wander when he looks at an object. If the parent gives a positive response to the second question, the child does not pass this screening. Such a response indicates that the child may have an eye problem.

Even though the child passes the other four tests of the battery, he is still referred through his parents to an eye specialist.

SIGNS OF EYE PROBLEMS. If the vision technician can observe that the child has any of the following eye problems, he does not pass this screening: strabismus, ptosis, nystagmus, or a difference in the size of the pupils.

FOLLOW-UP OF SCREENING

Follow-up of both school-age pupils and preschool children is an essential and necessary part of the health department's work. Public health nurses urge parents to take their children to an eye specialist. When the family is indigent, the nurse may need to assist in obtaining the child's examination through an eye clinic. The procedure differs slightly for school-age pupils and preschool children.

School-Age Pupils

After the vision screening program, the local public health department informs all parents of the results. When a pupil does not pass, the notification mailed to the parents includes a report form for the eye specialist to complete and mail back to the health department. The form, "Doctor's Vision Report — School," is reproduced here (page 197). If the form is not completed and returned within six weeks, a second letter is sent.

Telephone calls and home visits are made. Teachers, counselors, and even school principals assist in this endeavor.

The completed "Doctor's Vision Report" contains information concerning visual acuity, the defect, and treatment. Public health departments use information on the doctor's reports to assist in locating children who may be candidates for a program for the visually impaired. Children and young persons in the following categories are referred to special education departments for evaluation: those with nystagmus or cataract; young children who have a high correction for either hyperopia or myopia; and those with corrected visual acuity of 20/70 or less in the better eye, or even 20/50 if the child is in an early elementary grade.

Preschool Children

Parents usually bring preschool children to the screening site. As soon as a child completes the battery of five tests, parents are informed of the results. The results must be carefully interpreted to the parents; this includes mentioning the limitations of the screening procedure. When a child passes all the tests, parents are given a statement taken from the bottom part of the "Preschool Vision Screening Record" (p. 198). The statement is addressed to the school administrator and indicates that the child has passed, thus complying with the requirement of the Public Health Code.

When a child does not pass, parents must understand and be impressed with the importance of securing an eye examination for their child. As with school-age pupils, the parents are given a form for the eye specialist to complete and return to the department of health within six weeks. The form, "Doctor's Vision Report — Preschool," is reproduced here (p. 197). If the form is not completed and returned within the required time, a public health nurse contacts the parents, urging them to have their child's eyes examined, and offering other assistance, if needed.

RELATIONSHIP BETWEEN SCREENINGS AND REFERRALS

This relationship differs somewhat for school age and preschool children.

School-Age Pupils

The Vision Technician's Manual for Screening School-Age Children,
(1979, p. 8) states that of the children and young persons
screened, between 7 and 12 percent are referred to eye specialists. The percentage referred varies from one area to another.
Factors affecting referral rate are (1) grade and age levels, the
higher the grade and age, the more referrals; (2) frequency of
screening, the less frequent screenings, the more referrals; and
(3) socio-economic status of the area, the lower the status, the
more referrals.

The following is recent information* concerning school-age
pupils screened in Michigan:

> 1978-79   566,754 screened
>   45,967 or 8.1 percent referred
> 1977-78   580,694 screened
>   46,380 or 7.9 percent referred

Preschool Children

Between 5 and 10 percent of the preschool children screened
are referred through their parents to eye specialists. Local public
health departments report that the majority of children who are
then given professional eye examinations, are found to have
vision defects.

The following is recent information concerning preschool
and kindergarten children screened in Michigan:

> 1978-79   69,172 Preschool
>   3,758 or 5.4 percent referred
>   53,835 Kindergarten
>   123,007 Total screened
> 1977-78   69,296 Preschool
>   3,762 or 5.4 percent referred
>   49,224 Kindergarten
>   118,520 Total Screened

---

* The data from school and preschool screening are reported by Kenneth H. Mehr,
Assistant Chief, Vision Section, Michigan Department of Public Health.

FINDINGS FROM EYE EXAMINATION REPORTS

These findings concern only school-age pupils.

The Vision Technician's Manual for Screening School-Age Children, (1979, p. 8) lists the results and recommendations of the professional eye examination reports, with some children and young persons being in more than one category.

Glasses:	65 to 85%
Eye exercises:	5 to 10%
Medical or surgical treatment:	2 to 5%
Difficulty uncorrectable:	2 to 5%
Apparent difficulty; no treatment recommended at present:	3 to 10%
No apparent difficulty:	2 to 10%

RECOMMENDED FREQUENCY OF SCREENING

School-Age Pupils

The Vision Technician's Manual for Screening School-Age Children (1979, p. 7) makes the following recommendations with regard to frequency of screening: the complete Michigan battery should be given pupils every other year in grades 1, 3, 5, 7, 9, and 11; the Snellen Chart test for visual acuity should be administered to pupils during the even grades, 2, 4, 6, 8, 10, and 12.

Referral of pupils on the basis of observation, especially by teachers, should be a continuing process, even though screening procedures show vision to be within normal limits.

Preschool Children

The Vision Section of the Michigan Department of Health and eye specialists recommend vision screening once a year before the child enters school.

Some school-age pupils as well as preschool children who fail screening tests will be found by the professional eye examiner to have normal vision and healthy eyes. Such findings are to be expected. Parents, eye specialists, and others concerned with vision, should note the advice given by the National Society for the Prevention of Blindness.

If the examination shows no abnormalities, professional eye examiners must not interpret this as a waste of time and money but as valuable information and an important part of the child's total health care (Hatfield, 1979, p. 78).

REFERENCES

Blackhurst, Robert T. and Radke, Edmund. "School Vision Screening in the State of Michigan." *Sightsaving Review*, 1964, 34, 1-8.

Hatfield, Elizabeth M. "Methods and Standards for Screening Preschool Children." *Sightsaving Review*, 1979, 49, 71-83.

Jobe, Fred W. *Screening Vision in Schools*. Newark: International Reading Association, 1976.

Radke, Edmund and Blackhurst, Robert T. "Preschool Screening of Vision: The Michigan Experience." *Sightsaving Review*, 1978, 48, 99-105.

Vision Technician's Manual for Screening Preschool Children. Lansing: Vision Section, Michigan Department of Public Health, 1979.

Vision Technician's Manual for Screening School-Age Children. Lansing: Vision Section, Michigan Department of Public Health, 1979.

Chapter 11

EDUCATIONAL PROCEDURES FOR THE PARTIALLY SEEING

T HIS CHAPTER will be concerned with partially seeing or low-visioned children rather than blind. However, it should be noted that more than 70 percent of the blind children, those who use Braille and are enrolled in special programs for the blind, have slight amounts of vision. Their vision ranges from sheer light perception to about 10/200 visual acuity; that is, about 10 percent visual efficiency. All these children require assistance and encouragement to use their eyes to the fullest extent. They should have periodic professional eye care to help them retain and even increase their ability to see. Visual abilities improve with stimulation and use.

> Even a slight amount of vision allows the sense of sight to enter into the learning process of a child. (Hiltz, 1967, p. 503).

Partially seeing children are generally defined by the amount of useful vision they have. Their corrected visual acuity is usually 20/70 or less; that is, their visual efficiency is 64 percent of normal or less. Also, the Michigan code considers children partially seeing if their field of vision is restricted to no more than 20 degrees diameter. During recent years more children whose visual acuity is 20/200 or less (20 percent of normal vision or less) are being educated as partially seeing rather than blind. In addition, a few children, such as those with nystagmus, may have more than 20/70 corrected vision. Thus, there will be a wide range of visual acuity ratings among children considered partially seeing.

Certain low-visioned children are borderline so far as their method of education is concerned. When the child is ready for beginning reading and writing, it is difficult to determine whether he should be educated as partially seeing and use print or as blind and use Braille. In such instances, the special

165

teacher's observations and evaluations as well as the medical eye specialist's examination reports and recommendations, are the important deciding factors.

Low vision and its accompanying problems are much more of an educational handicap for some boys and girls than for others. Two children with exactly the same amount of vision may have very different reactions to their limitation. One may progress satisfactorily in the regular grades of the school. The other needs to be assigned to a resource room for the partially seeing where he will have much individual instruction and use special equipment. This difference between the two pupils can be attributed to such factors as ability to use the vision, motivation, concentration, and intelligence. The nature of the eye condition and age of onset certainly influence these factors as do family interest and support.

INVOLVEMENT OF THE HOME

Parents are usually the first to notice a visual defect, since most are evident before the child is two years old. They will have the child's eyes examined by a medical eye specialist and corrected to the greatest possible extent.

It is a well-known fact that the early years of a child's life have been shown by psychologists and educators to be a period in which intelligence develops most rapidly. Parents and other members of the family should help the child compensate for his visual deficiency by making certain that he develops a rich background of knowledge and experiences. Family cooperation and involvement are of utmost importance.

In many cities a preschool teacher-consultant makes home calls on children with very low vision. In Detroit the infants and preschool children are referred by doctors, nurses, social workers, hospitals, and by a county-wide network for locating impaired children, Project FIND. Some such children are able to develop at approximately the same rate as the normally sighted. The teacher-consultant discusses and demonstrates to the parents skills the child can achieve if given assistance and encouragement.

Examples of some of these motor and behavioral skills are:

holding the head erect, sitting with support and without, standing, creeping, walking, climbing stairs, inserting objects into holes, turning the pages of a book, using a crayon on paper to make circles or lines, stringing beads, nesting boxes, throwing a ball, using sound as an aid to locate and grasp an object, recognizing body parts, searching for the sound of a voice, listening to rhymes and jingles, retrieving and naming an object from a group of objects, removing clothing, and learning to dress. Examples of social skills are waving good-by, learning pat-a-cake, using a spoon and eating properly, and showing courtesy.

After working with the child for awhile, the consultant and parent develop an individual education program with both long- and short-term goals. Between the ages of two and three, if a child has very low vision, he and the parents make periodic visits to a preschool class for visually impaired children. These visits promote a smooth transition from home to regular school attendance in such a class. If the child's vision is not severely impaired, he and the parents would make periodic visits leading to regular attendance in a nursery school in his own neighborhood.

Conversation with the preschooler expands his oral and meaning vocabularies and helps him develop correct language patterns. When the child enters school and is taught to read, his rich background of firsthand experiences and skills will assist him in interpreting what he reads and in anticipating ideas. Expectations for developing the child's potential will replace the parental desire to overprotect him.

As the child progresses through school, parents can continue to assist and encourage him, for example, by reading aloud stories or some assignments. Another way is to demonstrate certain play skills to the child, such as jumping rope and roller skating, which sighted children learn from casual observation. It is almost a necessity for boys and girls at upper grade levels to have recorders and record players in their homes. Learning some of their lesson material and assignments through listening will enable them to assimilate more in less time, since many partially seeing children must expend real effort to distinguish reading material. This is particularly true as the child progresses to higher grade levels where fewer materials in large type are available.

EDUCATIONAL CONSIDERATIONS

The school should give the low-visioned child special consideration in certain areas. These include good physical condtions in the classrooms, certain special equipment, and attention to his vision. The school frequently needs to provide orientation and mobility instruction and typewriting lessons as necessary parts of the school curriculum.

Physical Conditions

Optimum physical conditions should be available. Many partially seeing pupils require higher levels of lighting than do other children. Adequate lighting which is well distributed and gives visual comfort is a necessity. Such lighting minimizes eyestrain and fatigue, while increasing the speed and efficiency of reading.

The luminance ratio between the task area and the surroundings should not exceed 3 to 1; that is, nothing in the background of the work and study area should be more than three times darker or lighter than the task itself. A dark spot or a bright spot in the working area is distracting and causes difficulty in focusing. The eye tends to focus on the bright spot.

There are a number of classroom features which can increase the reflectivity level in a classroom, and thus reduce the work-background contrast while making better use of the available illumination: mat-finish furniture that is light in color; ceilings with an 80 percent reflective factor; walls, including bulletin boards and chalkboards, with a 60 percent factor; and floors with a 20 to 30 percent factor.

There should be plenty of chalkboard area so that materials written by the teacher or children are not crowded but well-spaced. Sufficient electrical outlets provide for much use of audio and visual equipment. The physical arrangement of furniture, equipment, supplies, and books should be consistent. Books and materials should be stored in a definite place that is easily accessible. A well-ventilated room and comfortable temperature are conducive to work and study.

There should be an underlying system of efficiency and consistency, and some type of disciplinary control. Noise, whether from an outside or inside source, should be limited to a certain level. It is easier for low-visioned children, many of whom depend on their ears more than their eyes, to work in a quiet room.

Special Equipment and Supplies

Certain special equipment and supplies assist the child in making normal progress through school.

SPECIAL DESKS. Movable desks of various sizes enable partially seeing children to be in the center of class activities and in the best place in regard to lighting. Adjustable tops are essential. Some children require a desk top that adjusts to a 50 or 55 degree angle in order to bring the material close enough to the eyes for comfortable seeing and for good posture. Desk easels or reading stands sometimes must be substituted for the adjustable tops.

OFF-WHITE PAPER AND HEAVY PENCILS. The children should use off-white or buff paper of good quality. When young children use ruled paper, the lines should be widely spaced and the color contrast not too strong. Pencils with fairly soft, heavy lead make a broad, clear line, as do felt tip pens.

BOOKS WITH LARGE TYPE. Large type books are a necessity for many partially seeing children, especially for those in the elementary grades. Many basic readers and other books are now available in large type at these grade levels. Some children will be able to read standard type. However, no young child should be expected or encouraged to read print so small that he must be within 2 or 3 inches from the page in order to distinguish it. Such a procedure not only creates tension and discomfort but also greatly reduces reading speed and comprehension.

Those who select reading materials need to insure that they have clear type and illustrations, adequate spacing between lines, wide margins, and maximum contrast between background and type.

LARGE TYPE TYPEWRITERS. Beginning in grade four, typewriters with large size type are used by many partially seeing children. The type on these machines, together with heavily inked ribbons, enables children to read what they have typed.

Typewriters with standard size type are used by some students at the secondary school level. Electric typewriters should be provided, if possible, especially for younger children. The keys respond to the slightest touch and the carriage return is automatic. Along with the typewriters, adjustable typewriter desks and adjustable chairs are required; also, copyholders or stands that are adjustable vertically as well as horizontally.

RECORDING MACHINES. Dictating machines and records may assist in teaching typewriting and in doing assignments as do cassette players and tapes.

RECORD PLAYING MACHINES. Record playing machines present literature, history, and other materials. The Library of Congress gives nationwide service to the visually impaired through Talking Book machines and records as well as cassette players and tapes. The material available is essentially that of a public library, including best sellers, leisure time reading, and certain journals and magazines. The service can be obtained from regional depositories.

TELEVISION. Selected television programs have many advantages for the children. The use of films, pictures, maps, and other visual aids make school subjects meaningful.

Closed circuit television for magnification of material is a more recent development. The book or other material is placed under a TV camera while the enlarged print or material is viewed on the screen of the TV monitor. The high magnification and good contrast make the material readable for partially seeing students. Closed circuit television is especially helpful in middle and senior high schools where fewer materials are available in large type.

OPTICAL AIDS. There are a great variety of hand and stand magnifying aids available. Harley and Lawrence (1977, pp. 83-92) list, describe, and illustrate some of these. Magnifying aids that do not distort the material being read are important. Lack of distortion eases and speeds reading, enabling the pupils to read many books in regular type. Telescopic aids for viewing in the distance are helpful for older pupils. However, for younger children, such telescopic aids are hard to handle and the narrow visual field is frustrating to them.

Attention to Vision

When the low-visioned child enters the special program, the medical report from the eye doctor and the School Vision Clinic are sent to the special teacher. Thereby the child knows that his visual impairment is recognized and taken into consideration. His apprehension is replaced by a desire to accomplish and achieve. The special teacher will use the information on the report, as well as his or her own findings in regard to the child's vision, to adjust the program and instruction to the child's visual capabilities and to help other teachers recognize his visual status.

The teacher will explore the child's functional vision by various tests and activities. The confidence from such knowledge will enable him or her to proceed in a positive way. The teacher will know that many reading and curriculum problems are not associated with the child's low vision. In certain instances the teacher will decide by observation and evaluation which materials or objects a child is unable to see rather than suggesting to the child that he cannot see them.

It is only by using vision that its potential is realized. Whatever vision partially seeing children have should be strengthened in every possible way. When profitable, both near and far vision aids should be prescribed and used under the direction of an eye specialist. As a child progressively learns to interpret the images he sees and to increase his concentration, his visual functioning will improve. Instruction in the process of learning to see and in the use of visual aids must be very gradual since many children will need much help in learning to use the aids effectively.

Some children, particularly those in the lower age group, experience an improvement in vision after using their eyes for reading and other near-point activities. Other children will have an increase in visual functioning (though not in visual acuity), after they have received definite and intensive teaching with appropriate materials.

For those children who have such low vision that they see only broad outlines, the teacher will attempt to clarify their dim visual observations. This will be accomplished by extra help in visual discrimination, more explanations, and many firsthand experiences.

Some partially seeing children, frequently those with the lowest vision, may be superior in auditory perception and memory, because they have had to depend on their hearing more than do other children. In such instances the special teacher will encourage the continued development of auditory learning and memory while attempting to improve the visual potential.

The special teacher will observe how long a child can read or do other near-point activities without discomfort or fatigue. Also, the teacher will notice in which part of the room (the window side or wall side, for example) the child generally moves his desk in order to see and work most comfortably. By the time pupils have reached upper elementary grades, they should be given this information and know how to use it. In addition, the pupils should be taught some basic eye anatomy and physiology so that they will have a background for understanding their own vision problem, and how to use their eyes to the fullest.

Orientation and Mobility Instruction

The task of moving about is exceedingly difficult and complex for some partially seeing children with very low vision. They must expend real effort to see, and their vision may not be efficient in areas where the light is very dim or very bright.

> It is not uncommon for partially seeing children with very low vision to be misunderstood because of slow reactions or confused responses to some environments. In a brightly lighted, noisy cafeteria, a new classroom, or a room in which the furniture has been moved about, or on a sunny playground where running children and shadows blur and shift, for example, partially seeing children may have difficulty organizing their perceptions of what is around them. (Reynolds and Birch, 1977, p. 615).

Mobility instructors, with the assistance of special teachers and parents, can help partially seeing children become oriented to their environment and go from place to place with comparative ease. This is a gradual learning process for the child must first travel within a limited environment and then an enlarged one.

As the child meets the challenge of increasing his mobility, he gains self-confidence and poise. His ability to travel independently broadens his opportunities for extra-curricular activities and social functions at school and at home. As a high school graduate, the mobile student is not narrowly restricted in his choice of colleges to attend. As an adult, he has a much wider range of employment opportunities.

In Detroit those children who transfer from the preschool teacher-consultant service to a special prekindergarten program, receive the assistance of a mobility instructor. The children are taught to move about the classroom with ease, to find their own lockers, and to locate the drinking fountain. Physical fitness activities add to their mobility competence. The special teacher, physical education teacher, and parents follow through on suggestions given by the mobility instructor.

When these very low visioned children and others enter the program for the partially seeing, some continue to receive mobility instruction. The amount of instruction required is an individual matter and depends mainly upon the child's vision and how he uses it.

Some years ago a Detroit Mobility Evaluation Report was developed by special teachers in consultation with the mobility instructor and the supervisor. The report is addressed to parents and gives them a periodic evaluation of the child's accomplishments. The report has six sections: (1) posture and walking, (2) use of senses, (3) use of basic knowledge and concepts, (4) indoor mobility, (5) outdoor mobility, and (6) needs or inadequacies. The ratings are "S" for satisfactory, "N" for needs to improve, and "X" for not expected to accomplish at present. The report is signed by both the mobility instructor and the special teacher. It is reproduced on pages 201 through 204.

POSTURE AND WALKING. Posture and walking are improved by participation in physical education classes, especially physical fitness programs, and activities in which the child develops muscle tone, coordination, and skill in body movement. Swimming is a healthful sport which children enjoy. Many visually impaired children are given weekly swimming lessons at a YMCA during elementary school years. This instruction enables the children to participate in regular swimming classes and programs when they enter middle and high schools.

USE OF SENSES. This section emphasizes all the senses as avenues of learning. The instructor demonstrates how to make the pupil more alert to sounds, how to help him locate their sources, and how to sharpen the senses of touch, smell, and taste. The use of vision is included under this section. The pupil may learn to use a telescopic aid to locate a street name or house number, for example. Pupils who benefit from low vision aids are encouraged to go to a low vision clinic. Sometimes this trip is made with a group of children. However, it is preferable for parents to accompany their child to the low vision clinic.

USE OF BASIC KNOWLEDGE AND CONCEPTS. This section includes the understanding of measurements, shapes, and cardinal directions which many normally seeing children know from casual observation. Such information and concepts are more important for low-visioned children. They give meaning to the words they speak and impart confidence as they travel about.

INDOOR MOBILITY. By means of indoor mobility, the child is taught to travel within the school, learning directions and developing a cognitive map of the school. He learns to locate school entrances and exits, the office, fire drill routes, classrooms and their numbering patterns, and other important areas. A pupil who has learned to travel within the school, is permitted to do errands. This new responsibility is an important factor in developing self-confidence.

OUTDOOR MOBILITY. This section mainly concerns the partially seeing pupils who may need to use a cane for travel. At the middle school level the mobility instructor provides the pupils with outdoor travel instruction in the school neighborhood. The instructor must be certain the children understand such terms as "block," "intersection," and "traffic lanes," and how to cross large traffic intersections without depending on their vision to see traffic lights.

As the pupils travel outdoors, they learn the names of streets and bus routes, and how to locate various buildings and shops, such as a drugstore, bakery, and post office. They may visit a fast food restaurant, learn to order, and make change.

After the pupils become independent travelers in the school neighborhood, their instructor gives them lessons in their home community. The pupils are then taught to use public transportation, and they gradually learn to travel alone to school. This phase of outdoor mobility may require parent counseling by the mobility instructor and persuasion by the pupils themselves. Many parents are apprehensive about having their children travel alone in a large metropolitan area.

NEEDS OR INADEQUACIES. These include such needs as the need (1) to develop initiative to travel, (2) to be more independent, and (3) to learn necessary routes to school. A checkmark is put beside each item in this section if the child or young person requires extra assistance.

As with all parts of the school curriculum, the orientation and mobility skills of many partially seeing children must be continually measured to be certain that growth is taking place. The Mobility Evaluation Report rates progress in this area. In addition, the report promotes a closer school and home relationship.

Typewriting Instruction

Today throughout the country typewriting is considered an essential part of the curriculum for partially seeing children. Since the child does not have to use his eyes in typing, his speed of writing can equal or even exceed that of normally seeing children. Typewriting helps to eliminate the frustration the pupil may experience in writing script. It increases concentration and listening skills so that the child develops ideas of accuracy, speed, and neatness.

The majority of children who have reached the fourth grade are eager for the challenge which typewriting offers. By this time, the child has had much experience in cursive writing. Children at this grade level already have considerable knowledge of spelling, and typewriting will increase their spelling efficiency. Further, typewriting started at the fourth grade level challenges the child to enlarge his vocabulary, increases the desire to try original writing, and develops skill in letter writing. At the same time the pupil is learning definite, clear-cut rules of punctuation.

However, the time to begin instruction should be kept flexible. Some children are ready to type by the third grade, and a few children may not type successfully before the fifth grade. Lower than average intelligence, as well as poor muscular control and coordination, retard the development of readiness for typing.

Typewriters that have standard keyboards but large bulletin type and heavily-inked ribbons make the print clearly visible for most partially seeing children. Material to be copied is placed on a stand or copyholder, adjustable vertically as well as horizontally so that the text is at eye level and can be brought as near the child as needed. The children are provided with adjustable typewriter desks and adjustable chairs. Small children will need footstools. Such equipment assists the pupils in maintaining correct posture at the typewriter. Correct posture will do more than any other single factor to insure proper typing habits.

The special teacher should be equipped with a standard typewriting guide. By also consulting a guide for instructing the visually impaired, the teacher will quickly discover adaptations in procedures that are necessary. In Detroit an itinerant typing teacher travels to the different schools to give instruction to partially seeing children and guidance to their special teachers. Thereby the teacher can follow through on the typewriting instruction.

The following are some suggestions concerning instructional procedures:

1. The children should be introduced to the main parts of the typewriter as they have need of them.
2. Typewriting instruction should introduce new skills gradually. Explicit directions need to be given in order to make a definite impression on the child.
3. Daily instruction is given in order to insure steady progress. However, a practice period of 10 to 15 minutes may be long enough for beginners.
4. As soon as the child has learned a few letters on the typewriter, he is encouraged to use them in forming and typing words. When he has learned all the letters, he is ready to compose simple sentences and short paragraphs.
5. Typing from dictation increases skill in composing at the typewriter. Dictating machines and records are used by middle and high school students. Dictating machines are especially helpful for students who wish to increase their speed. In

addition, the dictating machine may motivate other pupils to increase their typing skills as well as their speed.

6. Copying passages in books provides practice material. Many children will use large type books. It is essential that the material be understandable to the child and within his reading ability.
7. Pupils need to know and use all parts of the machine. For example, as soon as a child can type a paragraph, he will use the tab bar or key for indenting.
8. At regular intervals, the teacher will give a test to determine the level of typing proficiency which each pupil has attained. The results of the tests give the teacher definite information as to the pupil's present skill and future need for practice.

Many pupils have typewriters in their homes. After the children have had approximately one school year of instruction, they are ready to type during out-of-school hours. Later as the pupils increase their skill and speed, they look forward to using the typewriter for many activities at home and at work after leaving school.

PRACTICAL SUGGESTIONS FOR TEACHERS AND ADMINISTRATORS

The teacher will find the following procedures and suggestions helpful in working with partially seeing children. These are:

1. A longer and more intensive reading readiness program is recommended for those children who evidence a general developmental lag. No child with defective vision should be pushed into reading too soon.
2. The rate of instruction should often be more gradual than for other children. The teacher may need to stay longer at each level of instruction before increasing the difficulty in order that the material will make a deeper impression on the child.
3. Schedules should be planned so that children, especially in the primary grades, are not required to do prolonged periods of reading or close eye work at their desks. A change

of eye focus from reading or writing to a chalkboard lesson or oral discussion is helpful for this purpose. Such a procedure will prevent undue fatigue and increase the child's interest and attention span.

4. All materials that are presented to the children should be large and well spaced. This includes the teacher's writing on the chalkboard and charts, and materials on bulletin boards.

5. Extra help may be needed in visual discrimination, especially in letters and words that look somewhat alike, for example, *n* and *m, now* and *how.*

6. Emphasis should be given to expressive oral reading as opposed to word calling. This is especially difficult for certain low-visioned children who must be very close to the book in order to see the words. Since this results in projection of the voice into the book, such children should read orally for an audience of only a few boys and girls. There are a number of methods of increasing expressive oral reading: the child will tell the story, or part of it, rather read it orally; he will tell a story as the teacher records it on a chart, then the child re-reads the story; listening to his own reading from a tape recorder will encourage the child to try to improve.

7. More time should be given to complete assignments or adjusted assignments. Partially seeing children usually do both oral and silent reading more slowly than do other children. In fact, the act of reading may take two to five times longer for the partially seeing than for the child with normal vision. This may be due not only to low vision, but to the use of the optical aid close to the eyes in order to magnify the text.

8. Opportunity should be given for the child to explore many kinds of reading material and different sizes of type. Contrast, leading, spacing between letters and words, and different styles of type influence the speed of reading. In addition to the large type basal books used in the classrooms, school and public libraries have many beautiful books on their shelves with full-page colored illustrations and often larger than standard print. Such books are certain to satisfy many partially seeing children.

9. Much motivation, praise and encouragement are needed in order to hold and promote the interest of the children, always emphasizing the ability rather than the limitation.

10. Emphasis should be given to the development of the children's listening skills and auditory learning by such means as reading stories and poems aloud to them, and by using recording machines and tape recorders. As the boys and girls progress through school, the mere quantity of material to be assimilated makes recording a necessity. In addition, the recordings relieve the pupil of possible fatigue resulting from reading for too long periods of time. Occasionally a child will scan his book as he listens to the record or tape. This procedure tends to reinforce his learning.

11. Emphasis should be placed on teaching the child to organize his materials so that they can be located quickly and efficiently. This is often difficult because of the large size materials that he uses. Also, the child should be taught to organize his papers so there is not too much written work or too many math problems crowded onto one page.

12. Periodic evaluation of achievement with regard to personal adjustment, eye condition, and curriculum is very important. This should be followed by changes in the child's program to correct the difficulties.

The partially seeing child has certain special needs that require attention. During preschool years the parents are actively involved in his preparation for school. They will discover and have corrected, as far as possible, his eye difficulty. Their help can be augmented by a preschool teacher-consultant's knowledge of skills to be acquired as well as supportive facilities available to the child.

When the child enters school, he will be prepared to take his place with other children. His program will be carefully planned and carried out. It will be evaluated at regular intervals. The program will give special attention to his visual potential and will reduce the effects of his low vision.

The goal of this educational program, beginning in the home and always involving the home, is never to focus on limitations but to emphasize the development of the child's fullest potential.

REFERENCES

Corn, Anne Lesley and Martinez, Iris. *When You Have a Visually Handicapped Child in Your Classroom: Suggestions for Teachers.* New York: American Foundation for the Blind, 1977.

Cruickshank, William M. and Johnson, G. Orville, (Eds.). *Education of Exceptional Children and Youth.* Englewood Cliffs: Prentice-Hall, 1958.

Dunn, Lloyd M. (Ed.). *Exceptional Children in the Schools.* 2nd ed. New York: Holt, Rinehart and Winston, 1963.

Hanninen, Kenneth A. *Teaching the Visually Handicapped.* 2nd ed. Detroit: Blindness Publications, 1979.

Haring, Norris G. and Schiefelbusch, Richard L. (Eds.). *Methods in Special Education.* New York: McGraw-Hill, 1967.

Harley, Randall K. and Lawrence, G. Allen. *Visual Impairment in the Schools.* Springfield: Charles C Thomas, Publisher, 1977.

Hiltz, J. W. "Education of the Child with Defective Vision." In Ophthalmologic Staff of Hospital for Sick Children, *The Eye in Childhood.* Chicago: Yearbook Medical Publishers, 1967, 503-18.

Jones, John W. *The Visually Handicapped Child at Home and School.* Washington: U.S. Government Printing Office, 1968.

Reynolds, Maynard C. and Birch, Jack W. *Teaching Exceptional Children in All America's Schools.* Reston, VA: Council for Exceptional Children, 1977.

VOCABULARY

ACHROMATOPSIA: Total color blindness.

ACCOMMODATION: Adjustment of the eye for seeing at various distances; accomplished by changing the shape of the lens through action of the ciliary muscle.

ADD: Additional plus lens strength of the bifocal part of eyeglasses.

AFTER-IMAGE: The visual impression which remains after the stimulation of the retina has stopped.

ALBINISM: A genetically determined deficiency of pigment in the iris, choroid, and retina.

AMBLYOPIA EXANOPSIA: Uncorrectible, reduced vision; usually caused by disuse of the eye rather than by an organic defect.

AMBLYOSCOPE: Instrument with the characteristics of a stereoscope; it presents slightly different pictures to the two eyes. Used in evaluating and treating subjects with stabismus.

AMETROPIA: General term meaning the presence of a refractive error of any kind.

ANGLE OF ANTERIOR CHAMBER: Junction between cornea and base of iris.

ANIRIDIA: Absence of the iris. A thin iris margin is usually present.

ANISEIKONIA: A difference in the image size or shape in the two eyes.

ANISOCORIA: Unequal pupils.

ANISOMETROPIA: A difference in the refractive error in the two eyes.

ANNULUS OF ZINN: Fibrous ring in the back of the orbit where the extraocular muscles, except the inferior oblique, originate.

ANOPHTHALMOS: Absence of a true eyeball; caused by failure of the eye to develop. Sometimes used to describe missing eyeball after surgical removal.

181

ANTERIOR CHAMBER: Aqueous-filled space between the cornea and the iris.

APHAKIA: Absence of the lens; usually the result of cataract removal.

AQUEOUS: Transparent, watery fluid that fills the anterior and posterior chambers.

ARACHNODACTYLY: "Spider finger"; a condition in which the fingers and sometimes the toes, are abnormally long. Occurs in Marfan's syndrome.

ASTHENOPIA (Eyestrain): The symptoms produced by ocular muscle fatigue caused by errors of refraction, upset of accommodation, or muscle imbalance.

ASTIGMATISM: Refractive error which prevents light rays from coming to a point or focus on the retina; caused by unequal degrees of refractive power in the various meridians of the cornea.

ATROPINE: A drug that causes temporary paralysis of accommodation and dilation of the pupil; used in examinations and treatment.

AXIS: Refers to the meridian in which astigmatism is oriented. Designated by Ax, x, or Cx.

AXON: A nerve cell process that is typically single and long, and terminates in short branches; conducts impulses away from the cell body.

BINOCULAR VISION: Normal, simultaneous use of both eyes to focus on one object.

BIPOLAR CELLS: Nerve cells in the inner nuclear layer of the retina which connect rods and cones with the ganglion cells. (The axons of the retinal ganglion cells make up the optic nerve.)

BLEPHARITIS: Inflammation of the margins of the eyelids.

BLEPHAROSPASM: Involuntary contraction of the orbicularis muscle of the eyelid; excessive blinking.

BLINDNESS: The ophthalmologist's definition is the inability to see. The usual or legal definition in the U.S.A. is corrected visual acuity of 20/200 or less in the better eye, or a visual field diameter of no more than 20 degrees in the better eye.

BLIND SPOT: Physiological or normal: small, oval, non-seeing area in the visual field corresponding to the area of the optic disc.

BULBAR: Referring to the eyeball.

BUPHTHALMOS: Large eyeball caused by infantile glaucoma.

CALCIFICATION: The deposit of calcareous material (lime or calcium) within organic tissue so that it becomes hardened.

CANALICULUS: Small tube that drains tears from the upper and lower puncta; the two canaliculi join to form a common canaliculus before entering the lacrimal or tear sac.

CANAL OF SCHLEMM: A circular channel at the junction of the cornea and sclera through which aqueous passes before going into the venous system.

CANTHUS: The angle, outer or inner, at either end of the eyelid opening.

CARUNCLE: A small, fleshy, elevated structure in the inner angle of the eyelids.

CATARACT: Opacity in the lens of the eye; may be partial or complete.

CHALAZION: Granulomatous inflammation and enlargement of a meibomian gland.

CHEMOTHERAPY: The treatment of disease by chemical agents.

CHIASM: Consists of the junction of the two optic nerves; provides for the crossing of the nasal fibers to the opposite optic tract.

CHORIORETINITIS: Inflammation of the choroid and retina.

CHOROID: The vascular middle coat of the eye located between the sclera and retina.

CHOROIDITIS: Inflammation of the choroid.

CILIA: Eyelashes.

CILIARY BODY: Portion of the uveal tract between the iris and the choroid.

COLOBOMA: A gap in one of the structures of the eye, usually due to congenital malformation, but may be result of trauma or operation.

COLOR BLINDNESS: Diminished ability to perceive differences in color; causes confusion in the red and/or green portions of the spectrum. Weston (1980) states that the confusion is not particularly between red and green; the confusion is in the different shades of red or green, or both. Greens are confused with various shades of gray, red with various shades of brown.

CONCAVE LENS: Lens having the power to diverge light rays; used to correct myopia. Also known as diverging, reducing, myopic, negative or minus lens; designated by the minus sign (−).

CONES AND RODS: Two kinds of light sensitive cells in the retina. Cones are sensitive to fine detail and to color and are located primarily in the central retina. Rods are sensitive to light, even of low intensity, but not to color, and are located primarily in the peripheral retina.

CONGENITAL: Present at birth.

CONJUNCTIVA: Mucous membrane which lines the eyelids and the anterior sclera.

CONJUNCTIVITIS: Inflammation of the conjunctiva.

CONVERGENCE: Turning the eyes toward each other, or simultaneous turning of the eyes inward.

CONVEX LENS: Lens having the power to converge light rays; used to correct hyperopia and to furnish additional power for reading. Also known as converging, magnifying, hyperopic, positive or plus lens; designated by the plus sign (+).

CORNEA: Anterior, transparent portion of the outer coat of the eyeball.

CORNEAL CONTACT LENS: A very thin lens that fits on the cornea.

CORNEAL GRAFT (Keratoplasty): Operation to restore vision by replacing a portion of opaque cornea with transparent cornea; may be full thickness or partial.

COVER-UNCOVER TEST (Cover Test): A method of determining the presence and degree of phoria or tropia by covering one eye, thereby eliminating fusion.

CROSS CYLINDER: A lens combining plus and minus cylindrical lenses of equal power with axes at right angles to each other; used for determining the amount and axis of astigmatism.

CROSS-EYE: Esotropia.

CRYOTHERAPY: A form of therapy which consists of the use of cold or freezing.

CRYSTALLINE LENS (The Lens): A transparent, biconvex structure suspended in the eyeball between the aqueous and vitreous. Furnishes the additional focusing power needed to bring light rays to a focus on the retina.

CUP, OPTIC: Depression in the center of the optic disc.

CYCLITIS: Inflammation of the ciliary body.

CYCLOPLEGIC: A drug instilled into the eyes that temporarily relaxes the ciliary muscle, thus paralyzing accommodation; the drug also dilates the pupil.

CYLINDRICAL LENS: A lens in the form of a segment of a cylinder. Has no refractive power in one meridian, the axis; its greatest refractive power is in the meridian at right angles to the axis. Its principal focus is a line, not a point. Used to correct astigmatism, and designated by the letters Ax, x, or CX.

DACRYOCYSTITIS: Inflammation of the lacrimal or tear sac; usually due to infection secondary to faulty drainage of tears.

DARK ADAPTATION: The ability of the retina and pupil to adjust to dim light.

DETACHMENT OF RETINA: A separation of the inner layers of the retina from the pigment layer.

DEVIATING EYE: The eye that turns (in or out, up or down) in strabismus, as distinguished from the "fixing eye."

DIATHERMY: Coagulation of tissue by heat such as used in retinal detachment surgery.

DILATOR MUSCLE: Radial muscle in the stroma of iris; dilates the pupil.

DIOPTER: Unit of measurement of the strength or refractive power of lenses or of prisms.

DIPLOPIA: Double vision; seeing a single object as two.

DISC, OPTIC (Nervehead): A nearly circular, light colored area at the back of the retina where the optic nerve leaves the eye. The only portion of the optic nerve visible with an ophthalmo-scope.

DIVERGENCE: Turning the eyes away from each other, or simultaneous turning of the eyes outward.

DYSCHROMATOPSIA: Partial color blindness; difficulty in distinguishing colors.

DYSTROPHY: An abnormal tissue change, often a hereditary degeneration.

ECCENTRIC FIXATION: A condition in which an extrafoveal area of the eye is used for fixation.

ECTOPIA LENTIS (Dislocation of the Lens): Subluxation of the lens, usually upwards or up and in, and bilateral. Commonly hereditary.

ECTROPION: Turning out of the eyelid.

ELECTRORETINOGRAM: A graphic record of the electric activity of the retina, used especially in diagnosing conditions of the retina.

EMMETROPIA: ("Sight in Proper Measure"); correct sight or focus.

ENDOPHTHALMITIS: Extensive infection of the interior of the eye.

ENOPHTHALMOS: Abnormal displacement of the eyeball backward into the orbit.

ENTROPIAN: Turning in of the eyelid.

ENUCLEATION: Surgical removal of the entire eyeball; also, traumatic removal.

EPIPHORA: The overflow of tears onto the cheek; usually due to obstruction of the lacrimal passages.

EPISCLERA: Thin layer of vascular, elastic tissue overlying the sclera.

EPISCLERITIS: Inflammation of the episclera.

EQUATOR: Imaginary line encircling the eyeball midway between anterior and posterior poles; of significance in surgical localization.

ESOPHORIA: A tendency of one eye to turn inward.

ESOTROPIA: An inward turning of one eye; convergent strabismus.

"E" TEST: A method of testing visual acuity; often used for preschool children and for those in the primary grades.

ETIOLOGY: The cause of a disease.

EXENTERATION: Removal of the contents of the orbit, including the eyeball and lids.

EXOPHORIA: A tendency of one eye to turn outward.

EXOPHTHALMOS: Abnormal protrusion or bulging of the eyeball.

EXOTROPIA: An outward turning of one eye; divergent strabismus.

EXTRAOCULAR MUSCLES: External muscles of the eye which move the eyeball.

EYESTRAIN: See Asthenopia.

FARSIGHTEDNESS: See Hyperopia.

FIELD OF VISION: The entire area that can be seen by the fixed eye.

FIXING EYE: The nondeviating eye in strabismus.

FLASH BLINDNESS: A visual disturbance resulting from an intense light source.

FLOATERS: Fine, opaque particles in the vitreous which can activate the retina by casting a shadow upon it.

FOCUS: The point where light rays are converged after passing through a lens. In ophthalmology, to accommodate.

FOVEA CENTRALIS: A depression in the middle of the macula where vision is most acute.

FOOT-CANDLE: Unit of illumination; 1 foot-candle is generated by 1 lumen on 1 square foot of surface.

FRONTALIS: Muscle in the forehead that elevates the eyebrows.

FUNDUS: The interior of the eye visible through an ophthalmoscope. Comprises the retina, optic disc, and those parts of the choroid and sclera visible through the pupil.

FUSION: Cortical integration of the images received simultaneously by the 2 eyes.

GALACTOSEMIA: A congenital disorder in which there is an increased galactose level in the blood due to inability to metabolize milk sugar.

GANGLION: A mass of nerve cells with a common function; especially applied to a collection outside the central nervous system.

GLARE: Scattered light that interferes with the focused retinal image, thus reducing visual acuity.

GLAUCOMA: A disease of the eye characterized by abnormally increased intraocular pressure, and its consequences.

GLIOMA: A nerve tissue tumor.

GONIOSCOPY: A technique of examining the anterior chamber angle with the aid of a special contact lens and magnification, a gonioscope.

GONIOTOMY: An operation for infantile glaucoma. Abnormal tissue in the anterior chamber angle of the eye is incised in order to permit the entry of aqueous into the canal of Schlemm.

GRANULOMATOUS: Composed of or characteristic of granulomas or granulation tissue.

HEMIANOPSIA: Blindness of one-half of the visual field of one or both eyes.

HETEROPHORIA (Phoria): A tendency of the eyes to deviate.

HETEROTROPIA (Tropia or Strabismus): A deviation of the eyes from the normal straight position. Both eyes are not simultaneously directed at the same object.

HIPPUS: Spontaneous rhythmic movements of the iris causing spasmodic variations in the size of the pupil.

HISTOPLASMOSIS: A serious parasitic infection, sometimes affecting the eye.

HOMATROPINE: A drug with shorter action time than atropine; used primarily in refraction.

HORDEOLUM, EXTERNAL (Sty): An acute localized infection occurring at the eyelid margin, in a lash follicle and the associated gland of Zeiss.

HORDEOLUM, INTERNAL: Infection of the meibomian glands.

HYDROPHTHALMOS: An enlarged eye caused by infantile glaucoma.

HYPEREMIA: Increased blood in any part of the body, resulting in distention of the blood vessels.

HYPEROPIA, HYPERMETROPIA (Farsightedness): A refractive error in which the focal point for light rays from a distant object is behind or posterior to the retina with the accommodation at rest.

HYPERPHORIA: A tendency of one eye to deviate upward.

HYPERTROPIA: An upward deviation of one eye.

HYPHEMA: Hemorrhage in the anterior chamber.

HYPOPYON: Accumulation of pus in the anterior chamber.

IMPLANT: A spherical prosthesis buried in the orbit to replace partially the volume of an enucleated eye. Also, may refer to an artificial lens replacement after cataract surgery. (Actually, an implant is any material inserted into regions of the body to be retained in the body.)

INTRACAPSULAR: Refers to cataract surgery in which the lens is removed with its capsule intact.

INTRAOCULAR: Within the eye.

INTRAOCULAR PRESSURE: The fluid pressure within the eye.

IRIDECTOMY: Surgery, usually for glaucoma, in which a small portion of the iris is excised.

IRIDOCYCLITIS: Inflammation of the iris and ciliary body.

IRIS: Colored, circular membrane suspended behind the cornea and in front of the lens. Perforated by the pupil.

ISHIHARA COLOR PLATES: A test for color vision based on the ability to see patterns in a series of multicolored plates.

JAEGER TEST: A test for near vision using lines of type of various sizes.

KERATITIS: Inflammation of the cornea.

KERATOCONUS: A conical protrusion of the cornea, with central thinning.

KERATOMALACIA: Softening of the cornea; may be found as a late stage of xerophthalmia, and in other corneal conditions.

KERATOMETER: An instrument for measuring the curvature of the cornea; especially useful for fitting contact lenses.

KERATOPLASTY: See Corneal Graft.

LACRIMAL: Pertaining to the structures that secrete or transmit tears.

LACRIMATION: The secretion and flow of tears.

LACRIMAL GLAND: A gland which secretes tears; located above the outer angle of the eye.

LAGOPHTHALMOS: Failure of the eyelids to close completely.

LENS: Glass or transparent material having two surfaces with both curved or one curved and the other plane. (See Crystalline Lens.)

LENSOMETER™: Instrument that measures the strength or

refractive power of spectacle lenses; this is a trade name. Other trade names for instruments with the same purpose are Refractionometer™ and Vertometer™.

LEVATOR (Levator Palpebrae): The muscle that raises the upper eyelid.

LIMBUS: Junction or transition zone between the cornea and sclera.

LUMEN: Unit of light energy.

LUXATION OF LENS: A complete dislocation or displacement of the lens.

LYSOZYME: Enzyme present in tears which inhibits the growth of certain bacteria.

MACROPHTHALMOS: An abnormally large eyeball.

MACULA LUTEA (Yellow Spot): Small, central area of the retina surrounding the fovea centralis. With the fovea the macula comprises the area of clearest vision.

MARFAN'S SYNDROME: A congenital mesodermal disturbance of hereditary nature. Common features include tall stature, long fingers and toes (arachnodactyly), and subluxation of the lens.

MEGALOCORNEA: An abnormally large cornea.

MEIBOMIAN GLANDS: Sebaceous glands within the tarsal plates of the eyelids.

MELANOMA: A tumor arising from pigmented tissue.

MICROCORNEA: An abnormally small cornea.

MICROPHTHALMOS: An abnormally small eyeball.

MINUS LENS: See Concave Lens.

MIOTIC: A drug causing constriction of the pupil.

MONOCHROMATISM: Total color blindness.

MONOCULAR: Referring to one eye.

MASCAE VOLITANTES: See Floaters.

MYDRIATIC: A drug causing dilation of the pupil.

MYOPIA: A refractive error in which the focal point for light rays from a distant object is in front or anterior to the retina with the accommodation at rest.

NASOLACRIMAL DUCT: Duct between the lacrimal sac and the nasal cavity.

NEARSIGHTEDNESS: See Myopia.

NECROSIS: Death of a cell or group of cells in contact with living cells.

NYSTAGMUS: Rhythmic involuntary movement of the eyeball; it may be horizontal, vertical, rotatory, or mixed.

OCCLUDER: A cover for one eye; frequently used with children to treat suppression amblyopia.

OCCLUSION: Obscuring the vision of one eye in order to force the use of the other; commonly used in amblyopia.

OD, R, RE: Oculus dexter (right eye).

OPHTHALMOLOGIST, OCULIST: A physician who is a specialist in diseases of the eye.

OPHTHALMIA NEONATORUM: Hyperacute, purulent conjunctivitis in the newborn.

OPHTHALMOSCOPE: Instrument with a special illumination system for examining the interior of the eye.

OPTIC ATROPHY: Degeneration of the optic nerve.

OPTIC CHIASM: Junction of the 2 optic nerves where the nasal fibers cross to the opposite optic tract.

OPTIC DISC: See Disc, Optic.

OPTICIAN: Technician who grinds lenses for eye glasses, fits them into frames, and adjusts frames to the wearer.

OPTIC NERVE: The nerve that carries visual impulses from the retina to the brain.

OPTIC NEURITIS: Inflammation of the optic nerve.

OPTOMETRIST: A nonmedical practitioner licensed to examine eyes, to prescribe lenses, and to give visual training.

ORA SERRATA: Anterior boundary of the retina.

ORBICULARIS: A roughly circular muscle that closes the eyelid.

ORBIT: Bony eye socket.

ORTHO: Straight.

ORTHOPTICS: Techniques used in the diagnosis and treatment of ocular muscle imbalances, and in the measurement and treatment of amblyopia.

ORTHOPTIST: A technician who gives exercises to those with ocular muscle imbalances; also, measures muscle functions, fusion ability, and treats amblyopia.

OMOSIS: The passage of a solvent through a membrane from a dilute solution into a more concentrated one.

OS, L, or LE: Oculus sinister (left eye).

OU: Oculi unitas (both eyes).

PALPEBRAL: Pertaining to the eyelid.

PANNUS: Infiltration of the cornea with vascular tissue.

PANOPHTHALMITIS: Inflammation of all the tissues of the eye.

PARTIALLY SEEING CHILD: A term generally used for educational purposes: a child who has a corrected visual acuity of 20/70 or less in the better eye.

PARS PLANA: Smooth posterior portion of the ciliary body.

PATHOGENESIS: The mode of origin and course of development of a disease.

PD: Interpupillary distance.

PERIMETER: An instrument for measuring the extent of the visual field.

PERIPHERAL VISION: Ability to perceive the presence, motion, or color of objects outside the direct line of vision.

PHLYCTENULE: A tiny ulcerated nodule of the cornea or conjunctiva.

PHORIA: See Heterophoria.

PHOTOCOAGULATION: Use of an intense light beam for sealing retinal tears and detachments and for certain other eye abnormalities.

PHOTOPHOBIA: Abnormal sensitivity to light.

PHOTOPIC VISION: Vision at daylight illumination; usually refers to cone vision.

PHTHISIS BULBI: Atrophic degeneration of the eye caused by severe infection or injury.

PILOCARPINE: A drug used in the treatment of glaucoma.

PINK EYE: Any condition of the conjunctiva accompanied by congestion; also, an acute, contagious, epidemic form of bacterial conjunctivitis.

PLANO: A lens having no correction.

PLEOPTICS: Orthoptic method with the purpose of disrupting eccentric fixation and establishing foveal fixation.

PLUS LENS: See Convex Lens.

POSTERIOR CHAMBER: Aqueous-filled space between the iris and lens.

PRESBYOPIA: Blurred near or reading vision caused by decreased elasticity of the lens; may be evident soon after age 40.

PRISM: A wedge-shaped piece of glass or plastic that refracts or bends rays of light toward its base. Incorporated in spectacle lenses to overcome ocular muscle imbalance or paresis.

PROTOPSIS: Forward protrusion of the eye.

PTERYGIUM: A condition in which a triangular membrane grows from the conjunctiva over the cornea.

PTOSIS: Drooping of the upper eyelid caused by paralysis of the third cranial nerve, the oculomotor.

PUPIL: The round hole in the center of the iris.

RECESSION: Operation for strabismus in which the insertion of a muscle is moved backward, thus decreasing its action.

REFRACTION: Two meanings: (1) The bending of rays of light in passing from one transparent medium to another of different density. (2) In ophthalmology, the determination of refractive errors of the eye and correction by prescriptive glasses.

REFRACTIVE MEDIA: The transparent parts of the eye having refractive power: cornea and lens.

RESECTION: Operation for strabismus in which the insertion of a muscle is moved forward, thus increasing its action.

RETINA: Innermost light-sensitive coat of the eye.

RETINAL DETACHMENT: See Detachment of Retina.

RETINITIS: Inflammation of the retina.

RETINITIS PIGMENTOSA: A hereditary degeneration of the retina, usually beginning as night blindness.

RETINOBLASTOMA: A malignant tumor of childhood which originates in the retina; congenital in origin and embryonic in structure.

RETINOSCOPE: An instrument designed for the objective determination of a refractive error. Has its own source of light for reflection through the pupil.

RETROLENTAL FIBROPLASIA: An abnormal overgrowth of the retina occurring in premature infants who have had too much oxygen.

RHODOPSIN: Light-sensitive pigment in the rod cells.

RODS: See Cones and Rods.

SCLERA: Tough, white covering which, with the cornea, forms the outermost, protective coat of the eye.

SCLERITIS: Inflammation of the sclera.

SCOTOMA: An area in which the vision is depressed or abolished, situated within the visual field, so that it is surrounded by a normal or less depressed visual field.

SCOTOPIC VISION: Vision at low levels of illumination, usually refers to rod vision.

SLIT LAMP: A combination microscope and narrow beam of strong light for examining the anterior portion of the eye.

SNELLEN CHART: Chart for testing central visual acuity; consists of lines of letters or numbers in graded sizes drawn to Snellen measurements.

SPHERICAL LENS: A lens that consists of a segment of a sphere; its refractive power is the same in all meridians. Used to correct hyperopia and myopia.

SPHINCTER MUSCLE: Muscle in the stroma of the iris which constricts the pupil.

SQUINT: See Strabismus.

STAPHYLOMA: Bulging area of the uvea into a stretched sclera.

STEREOPSIS: Visual perception of depth, or 3-dimensional space.

STRABISMUS: See Heterotropia.

STY: See Hordeolum, External.

SUBLUXATION OF LENS: A partial dislocation or displacement of the lens.

SYMPATHETIC OPHTHALMIA: Severe inflammation in one eye following traumatic inflammation in the other eye.

SYNECHIA: Adhesion, usually of the iris to the cornea (anterior synechia) or lens (posterior synechia).

TAPETUM: A layer of tissue in the choroid of certain animals which reflects light strongly.

TARSAL PLATE or TARSUS: Fibrous tissue that gives shape to the eyelid.

TONOMETER: An instrument for measuring intraocular pressure; important in detecting glaucoma.

TELESCOPIC LENSES: Special lenses for persons with much sight impairment. Consists of 2 or more lenses mounted in a spectacle frame with a short distance between them to form a sort of telescope.

TRABECULOTOMY: Operation which involves the incising of the trabecular meshwork for the relief of glaucoma. (Goniotomy is one variation used extensively for the treatment of infantile glaucoma.)

TRACHOMA: Chronic, contagious, and serious keratoconjunctivitis; runs a prolonged course.

TROPIA: See Heterotropia.

UNIOCULAR: Pertaining to or affecting one eye.

UVEA (Uveal Tract): The iris, ciliary body, and choroid.

UVEITIS: Inflammation of the uvea.

VISUAL ACUITY (VA): Detailed central vision as in reading or writing.

VITREOUS: Transparent gel that fills the space behind the lens.

XEROPHTHALMIA: Corneal breakdown characterized by keratinization of the epithelium, eventually leading to ulceration and perforation of the cornea; seen in Vitamin A deficiency.

ZONULAR FIBERS: The numerous fine tissue strands which comprise the zonule.

ZONULE: A sheet of tissue made up of numerous fine tissue strands which stretch from the ciliary processes to the equator of the lens, holding the lens in place.

ZONULOLYSIS: Dissolving the zonules, as with a solution of chymotrypsin, in order to facilitate the removal of the lens in cataract surgery.

REFERENCES

Gennaro, Alfonso R. et al (Eds.). *Blakiston's Gould Medical Dictionary.* 4th ed. New York: McGraw-Hill, 1979.

Havener, William H. *Synopsis of Ophthalmology.* 4th ed. St. Louis: C. V. Mosby, 1975.

MacNalty, Arthur S. (Ed.). *Butterworths Medical Dictionary.* 2nd ed. Boston: Butterworths, 1978.

Schmidt, J. E. *Paramedical Dictionary.* Springfield: Charles C Thomas, Publisher, 1969.

Thomson, William A. R. *Black's Medical Dictionary.* New York: Barnes and
     Noble, 1969.
Vision and Its Disorders. NINDB Monograph No. 4. Bethesda: U.S. Department
     of Health, Education and Welfare, 1967.
Weston, Horace L. Unpublished notes to the author, 25 p., 1980.

APPENDIX

DOCTOR'S VISION REPORT – PRESCHOOL

Ref. on:
    Vision   Muscle
    History   Other

Name_____ Age_____ Date_____

Address_____ _____ _____

                                                     (City or Town)   County

Vision: Uncorrected   R   /   L   /   ⌈ o.u.   /   ⌉
        Corrected   R   /   L   /   ⌊ if signif.   /   ⌋

Defect: Myopia_____ Hyperopia_____ Astig._____ Muscle_____ Other_____ None_____

Treatment: Glasses_____ Exercises_____ Medical_____ Surgical_____

        No Rx at present_____ Not Necessary_____

Further Treatment Recommended: Medical____ Surgical____ Exercises____ Other____ None____

        Return in _____Weeks _____Months _____Years

        Comments: _____

                  _____

             Signed_____ Degree_____

H-360-P 8/75   **Michigan Department of Public Health**

DOCTOR'S VISION REPORT – SCHOOL

Ref. on:
    Vision   + lens
    Muscle   Other

Name_____ School _____

Address_____ Date _____

Vision: Uncorrected   R   /   L   /   ⌈ o.u.   /   ⌉
        Corrected   R   /   L   /   ⌊ if signif.   /   ⌋

Defect: Myopia_____ Hyperopia_____ Astig._____ Muscle_____ Other_____ None_____

Treatment: Glasses_____ Exercises_____ Medical_____ Surgical_____

        No Rx at present_____ Not Necessary_____

Further Treatment Recommended: Medical____ Surgical____ Exercises____ Other____ None____

        Return in _____Weeks _____Months _____Years

        Comments: _____

                  _____

           Signed_____ Degree_____

H-360 1/75   Michigan Department of Public Health

County _____ Screening Location _____

PRESCHOOL VISION SCREENING RECORD

CHILD'S NAME_____ BIRTHDATE _____ AGE_____

(If other than given name is used, please indicate_____)   yr.   mo.

PARENT OR GUARDIAN'S NAME_____ TELEPHONE NO._____

ADDRESS_____ CITY_____ ZIP _____

BRIEF EYE HISTORY

		Yes	No

1. Has your child ever been examined by an eye doctor? _____ _____

   When?_____ Reason _____

2. Name of eye doctor _____

3. When your child is ill or tired, do his eyes appear crossed or does one eye wander when he looks at an object? _____ _____

DO NOT WRITE BELOW THIS LINE

I Visual Acuity

Both eyes	0 1 2 3	4 5 6
Right eye	0 1 2 3	4 5 6
Left eye	0 1 2 3	4 5 6

Passed	Failed

RESULTS

II Corneal Reflection   _____ _____

R   L

III Cover-uncover Test: Near

   Right eye movement   _____ _____

   Left eye movement   _____ _____

   Cover-uncover Test: Far

   Right eye movement   _____ _____

   Left eye movement   _____ _____

IV Eye History   _____ _____

V Symptom Referral   _____ _____

   State symptom(s)_____

Passed	☐
Referred on Test _____	☐
Failed, Not Referred	☐
Rescreen for Visual Acuity	☐

_____
Date of rescreening appointment

_____
Technician

_____
Date of screening

H-101-P 1-6-70

68-70—3344

ATTENTION PARENT:

Please present this statement when enrolling your child in school for the first time. According to the requirements of Act 282 every child will need a statement that he has passed the health department screening, or he will need an eye examination by a doctor.

To School Administrator:

_____ passed the health department preschool vision screening test.

_____   _____
Date   Certified Vision Technician

_____   _____
Location   Health Department Director

Please retain this statement with other health records of child.

MDP

EYE REPORT FOR CHILDREN WITH VISUAL PROBLEMS   **R L B**

E OF PUPIL_____ SEX _____ RACE_____
e or print)   (First)   (Middle)   (Last)

ESS _____ DATE OF BIRTH _____
          (No. and street)   (City or town)   (County)   (State)   (Month)   (Day)   (Year)

E_____ SCHOOL_____ ADDRESS _____

STORY

. Probable age at onset of vision impairment. Right eye (O.D.)_____   Left eye (O.S.)_____

. Severe ocular infections, injuries, operations, if any, with age at time of occurrence _____
_____

. Has pupil's ocular condition occurred in any blood relative(s)? _____   If so, what relationship(s)? _____

EASUREMENTS (See back of form for preferred notation for recording visual acuity and table of approximate equivalents.)

VISUAL ACUITY	DISTANT VISION			NEAR VISION			PRESCRIPTION		
	Without correction	With best correction*	With low vision aid	Without correction	With best correction*	With low vision aid	Sph.	Cyl.	Axis
Right eye (O.D.)	_____	_____	_____	_____	_____	_____	_____	_____	_____
Left eye (O.S.)	_____	_____	_____	_____	_____	_____	_____	_____	_____
Both eyes (O.U.)	_____	_____	_____	_____	_____	_____	Date _____		

If glasses are to be worn, were safety lenses prescribed in: Plastic_____   Tempered glass_____   *with ordinary lenses

. If low vision aid is prescribed, specify type and recommendations for use. _____
_____

. FIELD OF VISION: Is there a limitation?_____   If so, record results of test on chart on back of form.

What is the widest diameter (in degrees) of remaining visual field? O.D._____   O.S._____

E. Is there impaired color perception? _____   If so, for what color(s)?_____

CAUSE OF BLINDNESS OR VISION IMPAIRMENT

A. Present ocular condition(s) responsible for   O.D. _____
vision impairment. (If more than one, specify all
but underline the one which probably first caused
severe vision impairment.)   O.S. _____

B. Preceding ocular condition, if any, which led   O.D. _____
to present condition, or the underlined condition, specified in A.   O.S. _____

C. Etiology (underlying cause) of ocular condition   O.D. _____
primarily responsible for vision impairment.
(e.g., specific disease, injury, poisoning, heredity
or other prenatal influence.)   O.S. _____

If etiology is injury or poisoning, indicate circumstances and kind of object or poison involved. _____

PROGNOSIS AND RECOMMENDATIONS

. Is pupil's vision impairment considered to be: Stable_____   Deteriorating_____   Capable of improvement_____   Uncertain_____

. What treatment is recommended, if any?_____

. When is reexamination recommended?_____

Glasses: Not needed_____   To be worn constantly_____   For close work only_____   Other (specify)_____

Lighting requirements: Average_____   Better than average_____   Less than average_____

Use of eyes: Unlimited_____   Limited, as follows:_____

Physical activity: Unrestricted_____   Restricted, as follows: _____

FORWARDED BY EXAMINER TO:

Date of examination_____
Signature
of examiner _____Degree_____

Address _____

Name
If clinic case: Number_____of clinic _____

PREFERRED VISUAL ACUITY NOTATIONS

DISTANT VISION. Use Snellen notation with test distance of 20 feet. (Examples: 20/100, 20/60). For acuities less than 20/200 distance at which 200 foot letter can be recognized as numerator of fraction and 200 as denominator. (Examples: 10/200, 3/200). 200 foot letter is not recognized at 1 foot record abbreviation for best distant vision as follows:

HM	HAND MOVEMENTS
PLL	PERCEIVES AND LOCALIZES LIGHT IN ONE OR MORE QUADRANTS
LP	PERCEIVES BUT DOES NOT LOCALIZE LIGHT
No LP	NO LIGHT PERCEPTION

NEAR VISION. Use standard A.M.A. notation and specify best distance at which pupil can read. (Example: 14/70 at 5 in.)

TABLE OF APPROXIMATE EQUIVALENT VISUAL ACUITY NOTATIONS

These notations serve only as an indication of the approximate relationship between recordings of distant and near vision and point type sizes. The teacher will find in practice that the pupil's reading performance may vary considerably from the equivalents shown.

Distant Snellen	Near A.M.A.	Near Jaeger	Metric	% Central Visual Efficiency for Near	Point	Usual Type Text S...
20/20 (ft.)	14/14 (in.)	1	0.37 (M.)	100	3	Mail order catalogu...
20/30	14/21	2	0.50	95	5	Want ads
20/40	14/28	4	0.75	90	6	Telephone directory
20/50	14/35	6	0.87	50	8	Newspaper text
20/60	14/42	8	1.00	40	9	Adult text books
20/80	14/56	10	1.50	20	12	Children's books 9-1...
20/100	14/70	11	1.75	15	14	Children's books 8-9...
20/120	14/84	12	2.00	10	18 }	
20/200	14/140	17	3.50	2	24 }	Large type text
12.5/200	14/224	19	6.00	1.5		
8/200	14/336	20	8.00	1		
5/200	14/560					
3/200	14/900					

FIELD OF VISION.   Record results on chart below.

Type of test used:_____   Illumination in ft. candles:_____

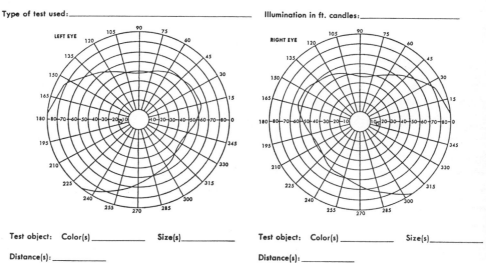

Test object: Color(s)_____ Size(s)_____   Test object: Color(s)_____ Size(s)_____

Distance(s):_____   Distance(s):_____

Stat 4 Rev/869/10M National Society for the Prevention of Blindness, 79 Madison Avenue, New York, N.Y. 10016

MOBILITY EVALUATION REPORT

DETROIT PUBLIC SCHOOLS   —   Special Education Department

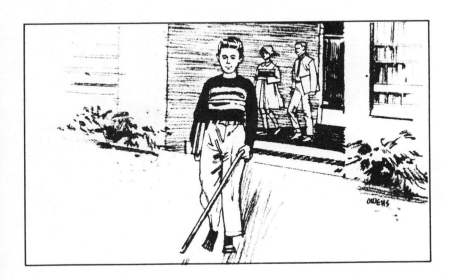

SCHOOL ------------------------------------

DATE ------------------------------------

NAME -- GRADE---------------

MOBILITY INSTRUCTOR---

TEACHER --

PRINCIPAL---

Superintendent of Schools

Posture and Walking

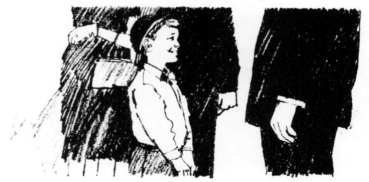

Stands and sits straight with head up.			
Faces person to whom he is speaking.			
Walks naturally with good posture and coordination.			

Use of Senses

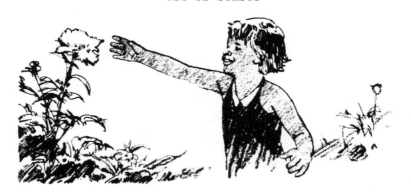

Is alert and uses senses well; not easily confused.			
Localizes and uses sound clues.			
Has good tactile sensitivity and memory.			
Makes good use of residual vision.			

Use of Basic Knowledge and Concepts

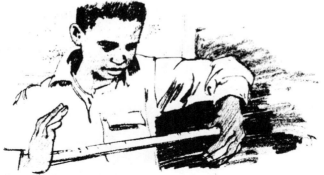

Understands measurements such as feet and yards.			
Understands shapes such as squares and triangles.			
Can repeat and follow a set of verbal instructions.			
Knows directions and can orient himself to them.			

Indoor Mobility

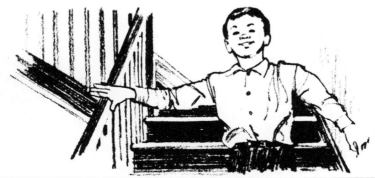

Walks about the room with ease.			
Can find materials in his desk and in the room.			
Knows how to find his locker.			
Can go to and from the lavatory without help.			
Travels safely on stairs.			
Knows the necessary routes in the school building.			
Shows initiative in traveling alone.			

Outdoor Travel

Is ready for cane travel.			
Can cross a street with or without a traffic light.			
Knows directions and street names in his neighborhood.			
Knows the route to school.			

Needs or Inadequacies

Appears to need an orthopedic evaluation.			
Needs to develop initiative to travel.			
Should be more independent — relies on guides too much.			
Needs to develop judgment of distances, sizes, textures.			
Should learn protective techniques for indoor travel.			
Should carry a cane as a protective measure.			
Needs to master basic cane techniques.			
Should learn necessary routes to school.			

Explanation of Marks

S	—	Satisfactory
N	—	Needs to Improve
X	—	Not Expected to Accomplish Yet

Parent's Signature

INDEX

205